STRONG
TO
SAVE

STRONG
TO
SAVE

YOUR GENX IMPERATIVE TO DIE HARDER AND LATER

DAVID EMERSON FROST

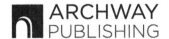

ARCHWAY
PUBLISHING

Archway Publishing books may be ordered through booksellers or by contacting:

Archway Publishing
1663 Liberty Drive
Bloomington, IN 47403
www.archwaypublishing.com
844-669-3957

ISBN: 978-1-6657-5271-8 (sc)
ISBN: 978-1-6657-5272-5 (hc)
ISBN: 978-1-6657-5273-2 (e)

Library of Congress Control Number: 2023921470

Print information available on the last page.

Archway Publishing rev. date: 01/24/2024

Health Disclaimer

"Strength training rewards us with lower fitness ages. I'm 48 in calendar years and I'm beating some athletes in their 20s."

Todd Vogt, Elite Para-athlete despite his early onset of Parkinson's Disease

Contents

Acknowledgments

Labors of love like this specialty non-fiction work - **Strong to Save** - are rarely solitary efforts. Mine certainly wasn't.

I extend my sincere apologies to my many mentors, coaches, and role models I missed in this short list of credits. I am truly grateful to each one.

I am particularly grateful to my New England forebears like Ralph Waldo Emerson, my parents, and strong family members. Many ancients stoics and modern practitioners contributed to this fit map as a body of knowledge.

I'm grateful to my wonderful wife Mary and to my collegiate rowing coach Carl Ullrich, who was of the greatest generation known to mankind and was a Marine's Marine. Our two incredible kids helped shape the worldly views that I share in this book.

Thanks to my artist, Austeja, and my writing coach, Hudson.

To Todd Vogt and Michael Brake and my many wellness and fitnes clients - particular thank yous are fitting!

I am awed, inspired by, and thankful for all those challenged athletes who keep on walking through hell.

I thank Uncle Sam and our many extraordinary soldiers, sailors, airmen, marines, and guardsmen plus their dependents, who serve our country and flag everyday.

-   Writers and military retirees like me appreciate the lifestyle and restful sleep that is made possible by those guarding over us.

And I thank YOU for changing your life with strong habits to serve others. There is no alternative.

Dave Frost

Foreword

I love lifting weights. I've been called a gym rat many times for doing my deadlifts, box jumps, and pullups. These sessions make me feel like a kid again, jumping and throwing stuff around or just moving heavy stuff like my crew coach's motor launch.

Lifting weights is a simple yet premier way to change this body of mine. Strength training makes me look better, helps me to feel great, and to perform at my best.

My serious strength training has made me become a faster rower and it's also helped me remain relatively injury free. My regular strength training lowers my "fitness age."

- ✓ I'm 48 in calendar years and I'm beating athletes in their 20s.
- ✓ I hold world records in rowing for my age and physical classification.
- ✓ Most importantly, my GenX resistance work helps me deal with my early onset Parkinson's Disease (PD) that was diagnosed 5 years ago. I had no alternative other than to stay **Strong to Save** with this challenge. After coming to grips with what life handed me, I first rowed and lifted for health and fitness. Then I started competitive racing again.

I earned a spot on the USA Paralympic Team for the 2019 World Rowing Championships in Austria. Recently, my crew mate and I finished second in the world championships in September 2023. Next, I will represent the USA at the 2024 Paralympic Games in Paris, France. *Citius, Altius, Fortius.*

Another great thing about strength training is that there are so many options and so few valid excuses. One can get a good strength workout in almost any environment, and in a short time, if you get creative as I hope you will.

Ladies and gentlemen, What is my challenge to you as a fellow GenX?

✓ Grab some free weight dumbbells, hit the leg press machine, or do some bodyweight pushups to lower your "gym age." You'll thank me as you down age to stay **Strong to Save** and Die Harder.

TV

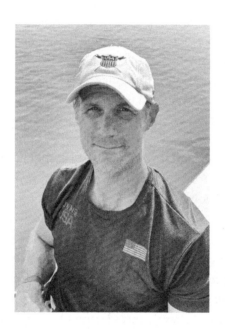

About Your Author

David E. Frost is an NFPT-certified master fitness trainer, with specialty certifications for weight loss and gluteal training. He is a rowing coach, a champion competitor, and an award-winning adjunct professor. After completing decorated careers in the US Navy and the business world, he founded Well Past Forty, LLC to promote health spans and lifespans for folks in their *middle ages* and *beyond*.

He specializes in nutrition, endurance, and strength training—adapting sessions for people dealing with cancer, MS, PD, CP, diabetes, and metabolic syndrome. He volunteers as a coach for underserved youths and military veteran Freedom Rows projects.

David earned his bachelor of science degree from the US Naval Academy and his master of systems management degree from the University of Southern California, focusing on human factors. He also studied at the Naval War College and the National Defense University.

Leveraging his professional certifications and continuing education, Dave provides group and one-on-one training sessions for athletes of all ages, helping them to add life to their years and to add years to their lives. He has written dozens of professional articles about practical and effective health span and lifespan boosters for athletes of all ages. He regularly appears on podcasts as a subject matter expert.

His personal achievements and awards include an Eagle Scout badge, a Technology Achievement award from Lockheed Martin Corporation, an Outstanding College Athlete of America (1975) award, Naval officer medals and commendations from our nation's Cold War days, USNA's Rusty Callow Award for dedication and leadership, and a 2016 Distinguished Faculty Award from the University of Phoenix. He has won the World Indoor Rowing Championships for his age group twice and has helped his crews win tens of National regatta medals.

A Vermonter by birth, David currently lives in San Diego with his wife, Mary. They celebrate two wonderful adult kids and three grandkids. He home-brews IPAs and Irish stouts to enjoy on weekends.

In 2019, his writings about twenty-first-century knowledge workers became a chapter in *Advances in the Technology of Managing People: Contemporary Issues in Business and Education.*

In 2020, Dave self-published his first specialty nonfiction book, *KABOOMER: Thriving and Striving into Your Nineties. KABOOMER* was a recent Firebird Award recipient.

Learn more about David and his work during and beyond his middle age at https://wellpastforty.com or at https://strongtosave.com.

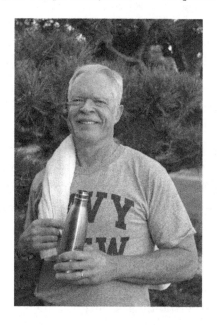

Introduction

"Even at age forty-one, I still hate losing (yet) setbacks have an upside; they fuel new dreams."

—Dara Torres, GenX Olympic champion, and author of Age Is Just a Number

"If something stands between you and your success ... move it."

—Dwayne "the Rock" Johnson, a very strong GenX

"I'm 48 in calendar years and I'm beating others in their 20s."

—Todd Vogt, an elite GenX Paralympian

Fuel new dreams, move it, beat others. Physical and mental strengths fueled Dara to overcome her setbacks. Strength shaped big parts of the Rock's enduring success. Both of their iconic lives of physical power, boldness, and resolve should inspire you to get physical, be bold, and stay resolute. Todd Vogt, as a third paragon of GenX performance, wrote the foreword to this book. Rowing is a challenging sport in multiple ways. Just imagine performing at elite world levels in this grueling sport. Then add an early onset of Parkinson's disease (PD) and you find a great GenX.

Dara, Dwayne, Todd—and *you* in Generation X (hereafter called GenX)—plan powerful and productive second halves of life. Here are your first two planning prompts:

- What *dreams* will you achieve after halftime?
- What things will you *move* to make your next fifty or so years your *best* years?

Strength, or "that on which anything is founded," is a true *cornerstone* of your healthy physical bank account. Strength is a most powerful personal asset. It is great to find and keep yours. Anything else in your life depends on it.

GREAT, GOOD, OR DECENT

Which of these 3 descriptors of GenX strength fits you? Soon you will soon learn what great, good, and decent powers mean to your health span and lifespan. Your bottom line?

A great GenX "down ages" while a decent GenX ages too soon.

Speaking of life and health, researchers determined in the worst COVID-19 pandemic years that the value of each human life was ten million US dollars. Yes, you are worth "7 figures." Take pride in your physical bank and stand strong as an enduring ten-million-dollar person. Invest in your physical bank as do Dara, Dwayne, and Todd.

Leverage these physical banking pages and weighty words for good reason. As The Town Pants sing, "words on a page can weigh a ton." Weigh these words to m*ake health* your new *wealth.* Move things in your way rather than skirt them. Invest in your cornerstone of functional strength for a notable return that is measured in extra years.

Why not Die Harder and Later?

Successful strength habits in *Strong to Save* are *science–backed* and *sweat-proven.* Think of these resource-packed pages as your "fit map" to become a *sthenic* symbol for others. You will read more strange-sounding terms in this fit map*.

Sthenic means *sturdy* and *strongly built.* Sthenic defines Dara, Dwayne, and Todd. I truly hope that sthenic will define you too. So, why not show and tell? Why not look great, act great, and perform great deeds in your GenX activities of daily and nightly life?

*Note: When you find a strange word or term like *musculus, biceps femoris,* or *latissimus dorsi,* please dog-ear that page and highlight that key word or phrase. Take comfort that a glossary of all terms, acronyms, and accepted abbreviations precedes the back cover of Strong to Save. Here is a first key term for both your glossary and motions.

PSOAS I WAS SAYING

This strange term, psoas, is a linchpin for your physical bank. Think of your psoas muscles as physical bank tellers that open up for business.

Each *psoas* is a *tenderloin* muscle anchored deeply above each hipbone and extending upward to your spinal column. Yes, the old word root of psoas is loin. Your two psoas muscles connect your body's upper and lower halves.

Your psoas are unique as linchpins! Some yoga practitioners call your psoas the "muscles of your soul." Think about that. You can call psoas your hip flexor muscles, as they are major contributors of flexion of your hip joints. There have been times when a psoas is a pain, whatever its hidden shape. You too may have *been there and done that* with soreness or pain. Either under-training or over-training those flexors may lead to such core symptoms. Be a student of your worthy endeavor to avoid or minimize psoas pain. Your healthy recipe to do that is your just-right strength training and stretching.

BE ON THE ALERT

You will see and read special fit map callouts named *Flex Alerts*. These *flexors* should shape your physical portfolio and trigger your sense and respond actions. Dog-ear or highlight these trusty callouts when you see them. Here's your first callout:

A great GenX can gain an extra *decade* of health span with strength work, restorative sleep, and good sustenance. This is your bank's triple crown, your trifecta. Think about ten added years without polypharmacy or physical malady. Get strong. *Power up* for ten added healthy years. You will read my terms of *down age* or *downaged* often in this fit map. Why? When you look, feel, and perform as one ten years younger than you, you are a **great downaged GenX**. Get down on invested implications of these weighty words.

Your down age efforts *offset* senescence (aging) and sarcopenia (which is age-related loss of mass and strength of skeletal muscle).

You naturally gain strengths and capitalize on your ten-million-dollar corpus.

GREAT!

Yes, nearly everyone in your generation has innate potential to pursue greatness. When I use the descriptor **great,** I mean performance that is notable, near faultless, and exceeding the norm of others.

Great *doesn't* mean super-sized or Brobdingnagian or herculean. Rather, *great* means that you keep on keepin' in as if you were ten years younger. *Can you think of any downsides for great functional strengths of youth?* If you can, I will eat my sweaty workout hat.

Yes, you can overcome adversity, as did Dara and Todd. Yes, you can gain functional strengths as you get older—yet not get old. But wait, wait...your GenX exercise can also improve Sexercise for your lover or mate and for you. As Dwayne Johnson might quip about animal spirits, why not love me as a rock?

You might ask this valid question, "Is *Strong to Save* for me?"

Strong to Save was written for you as a *great* member of "middle age." Think of yourself as a real-life action figure born between the calendar years 1965 and 1984.

As one of my ideal readers, *you* are passionate. You are knowledgeable. You are a student of your endeavor. You turn pages of this fit map to learn and perform habitually. You gain and retain cornerstone qualities of strength.

You will commit to bullet-proof action steps. Repeat after me. I will:

- *Make my next years my best years.*
- *Move stuff as my very good medicine.*
- *Be stronger to die harder and later.*

GRAVE CONSEQUENCES

Who wants to die *easier* and *earlier*?

I kid you *not*. As a powerful sign of our times, folks with strong grip strengths did *not* get sent to intensive care units for their COVID-19 illnesses. Dwell on that timely *die harder* medicine, please. Your cornerstone functional strength matters. Your strengths can be lifesaving!

Powerful themes of your strong fit map are offered in the call-to-action graphic, Figure I.1:

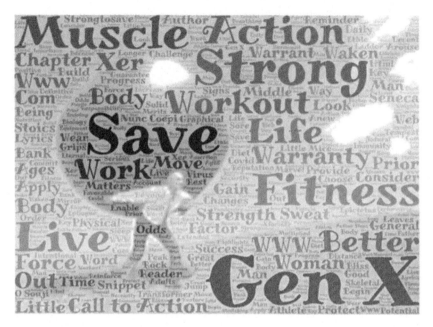

Figure I.1 Your Strong to Save themes

I add just one more introductory item before you dial up Chapter 1.

STAY TUNED

You will read about a radio station – WIFM – that is your personal down age station. This station fully addresses:

What's In it For Me?

Don't touch that dial…You probably haven't heard a certain seafarer's hymn on SiriuxXM™ or Spotify™. Or, you might have heard this hymn if you served in America's navy or are seated in a church pew. That certain seafarer's hymn, *"The Navy Hymn"*, is to be played on station WIFM at my funeral. *Yet that will have to wait because I am down aging as you will.*

One poignant phrase in that mighty hymn, namely "strong to save," became the title of this work, your fit map.

Strong to Save is a "source code" of this mariner's poem-turned-hymn by William Whiting in 1860. Whiting knew of and wrote lyrics about true hardships that mariners faced and overcame. He knew how sailors cleverly skirted danger and prevailed against wind and waves. He penned in his verse how seafarers used their brawn and brains to bring ships safely back to port.

Times may change, yet some ideals tapping brawn and brains do not. Again, strength means *that on which anything is founded*. Whiting's ideals for iron men (and women) are anchored sources for your cornerstone efforts.

Take just a moment to reflect on what enabling strength means in your physical bank. With strengths to save, you can:

1. Extend your own limits and offset both sarcopenia and senescence (i.e., move heavy stuff and move yourself as Socrates implored in antiquity.)
2. Keep calm and be ready to face danger's hours, COVID-19, emergent challenges, life's speedbumps and more.
3. Move the world in your longer and better life.

WIFM IS A BIG DEAL.

This powerful station is a big deal. Its sounds serve as great lifestyle drivers for you, and here is why...

Many of your generational peers, as decent GenX, will sadly experience a difference of many years between their health spans and lifespans. As a fact, and in this study, "many" is calculated as a percentage of negative *20*. So, if a decent GenX makes it to 85 years as lifespan, up to *17* of those years will be unhealthy. A decent GenX health span of only 68 years doesn't appeal to you or me. Oy!

It *is* a big deal to be vibrant for a decade or longer than a decent

GenX. Then "many" unhealthy years can be *reduced* to a value of almost zero. Here today in a healthy way, then gone tomorrow is much better for WIFM listeners like you.

Know your odds. Do your darndest to beat those odds for your generation's conditions, diseases, and comorbidities. Here is the weighty punchline:

A great GenX will have a very long healthspan. The length of that healthspan is very close to its ultimate stretched lifespan. A great GenX has a very good chance to become a healthy centenarian. Yup.

Living long and prospering certainly beats your alternative of a scoring a negative 20. Here's your second flex alert to codify your current strength:

FLEX ALERT #2:

- GenX females in their fifties should perform seven to ten push-ups and fifteen to nineteen sit-ups (crunches)—with solid form—to be classified as good. Yes, you can trust the Mayo Clinic on these flex ratings.
- GenX males in their fifties should perform fifteen to nineteen push-ups and twenty to twenty-four sit-ups (crunches)—with solid form—to be classified as good for functional strength.

Note: Body weight benchmarks like these are perfectly fine. When heavy stuff is not available to move, bodyweight exercises like pushups and crunches suffice. Now, shift performance standards for strength from good to *great*.

GREAT REDUX

Ladies and gentlemen, great folks in GenX can perform these strength sets for push-ups and crunches as if they were *ten years younger*. This means that someone aged at fifty calendar years performs as if *forty* in calendar years. Likewise, a great GenX at sixty calendar years is downaged to fifty fitness or gym years. Viva la difference!

- I leave details of how many *extra* pushups or sit-ups this down aging means for you as your first homework. Be an "A" student of your strong endeavor. Hint – start your homework with a professional weblog I authored for the National Federation of Professional Trainers @ https://www.nfpt.com/blog/fitness-age-older-clients.

La difference shapes a very fine investment for your physical bank. Thank you, Mr. Whiting, for this book title's source code and strong verse. Thank you, Dara, Dwayne, Todd, and thank you Socrates. I mention Socrates because Stoics of Ancient Rome and Athens had much ado about strength as an element of virtuous, well-lived lives.

An important highlight: Socrates and his peers believed that disabled people could recalibrate their lives by focusing on what they could achieve, rather than on what they couldn't achieve. One Stoic named Epictetus pressed on after he became physically disabled in his adult life.

As an adaptive coach and trainer, I include those in GenX who may be disabled or classified as challenged athletes. For my *Strong to Save* readers with physical or medical challenges, I exhort you to aim high, like Todd Vogt does each day, every training day. Yes, you can thrive and strive by achieving what you can, even when life has dealt you a "bad hand." Play that hand as best you can. As you will reaffirm on your journey, there is no alternative (TINA).

This acronym, TINA, recently arose in finance when stock prices were a tiptop investment in the longest bull market in our history. TINA, as a strong-to-save mantra, is a sthenic term for your physical bank too.

Should you, dear reader, already be in good standing for strength, then press on to become great. Should you be a tad delinquent in your strength measures as a decent GenX, then you should work to die harder and later as a good or great GenX.

One minor point: the fifty muscles used to frown do *not* count toward your habitual strength. Conversely, humor and a smile's muscle motion *do* count. Keep this in mind – the motions and exercises that please you are your best ones.

Please dwell on these two *Strong to Save* illustrations. Figure I.2 captures compelling WIFM concepts by the letter, and Figure I.3 reinforces your *Strong to Save* themes by numbers that truly count.

It is high time to get you started on your odyssey, whatever headwinds, and rough seas you face.

"Let's get it on," as Marvin Gaye once sang. TINA.

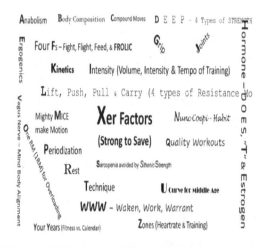

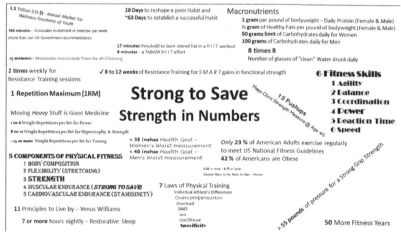

Kinetic Counts

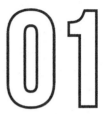

> "Physical strength is the most important thing in life.
> That is true, whether you want it to be, or not."
>
> **—Mark Rippetoe, author, and strength training coach**

S trength is your important truth for great GenX healthspan; and I want you to want it. This chapter will help you get a healthy grip on actionable numbers that count for strength and life.

Five *kinetic counts* follow. These numbers matter whatever your functional strength is and however your physical banking is today. Five is your golden rings number. You must move stuff in these five ways: 1.) lift, 2.) push, 3.) pull, 4.) twist, or 5.) carry.

This word, *kinetic*, simply means motion, or to put something in motion, as Dwayne Johnson and Mr. Whiting assert. And away you go to improve your physical strength, healthspan and lifespan by working these kinetic counts.

TINA, and that is a singular truth.

ONE TRUTH

Number 1: be stronger to die harder and later. Grip those introductory words of strongman Mark Rippetoe. May I paraphrase what he contends? The essential cornerstone of your physical bank is functional strength. You want and need to move and put things in motion for the next ~ fifty years. I'm not clairvoyant, so I cannot see into the future of 2073 AD. Yet, I can envision *you* as a naturally lean and strong outlier for GenX many years from now. Whether you want it to be or not, strength improves your health span and can help you move the world for much longer than can your peers.

1. Will you dodge the intensive care unit when others cannot because you have a "vise grip"? Yes, you can.
2. Will you experience a revved-up metabolism with lean skeletal muscle? You betcha.
3. Can you protect joints from injury? Yes.
4. Will you maintain an independent lifestyle for *a decade* longer than many of your peers? Yup.
5. Will you enhance your prospects to become a healthy centenarian? Very likely.

There is a corollary for these health and physical wealth codes. That corollary is: your own strength program is unique. *You* are one unique athlete, so your physical training and activities should correspond with your unique enablers. Don't just emulate another's resistance work. Be a student of your endeavor to choose what works for you on your journey. Now, double up …

TWO AGES—YOUR FITNESS AGE AND CALENDAR AGE

#2: The stronger you become, the greater are the performance differences between your fitness or gym years and your calendar years on this zany planet.

✓ Shoot for a downaged difference of ten (!) years.

I kid you not. Neither does Mark Rippetoe. I commend to you his book, *Practical Programming for Strength Training*, or *PPST3*. You can and should take his proven lessons about safe, rewarding strength training to your own physical bank. There is no doubt that strength is a cornerstone of your performance for decades to come. Remember that restorative sleep and clean sustenance also help you build your returns on investment.

You will learn about four types of cornerstone strength to bank in a bit. In the meantime, may I offer a quick thought about "my" industry of fitness? I do not disparage "big box" gyms or fitness clubs. (I started my own personal trainer career in such a big box.) Yet, Rippetoe suggests that it can be a challenge to improve your fitness age in those establishments. That is a shame. Do not be shamed. Your strength training requires time to do your regimens, to follow safe instructions, and to focus on your unique training goals. Work these sthenic imperatives of yours, wherever you are, in a big box or home garage. Work against resistance—in five ways—two or three times weekly until you are ninety in calendar years and correspondingly eighty in downaged fitness years.

Your number 2 also represents the average time in minutes that a committed GenX will devote to self-myofascial release (SMR) of tight muscles and connective tissue. *Do not* underestimate the utility of releasing tight fiber to down age and to perform better. *Do* invest those few extra minutes to help your body respond. Note: a full fit map of dynamic and static stretching, plus SMR and proprioceptive neuromuscular facilitation techniques is beyond the intended scope of Strong to Save. A professional article that I wrote about stretching skills (https://www.nfpt.com/blog/senior-stretching-skills) is one resource to help you become a better student of stretching. I devoted a whole chapter of KABOOMER to proper stretching, so that is another resource for you. I ask clients to think of proper stretching and release techniques as "flexible" investments in their physical banks.

This number two also suggests a buddy workout, or a 1+1 workout between a personal trainer and her/his client. Yet, as one rock group sang, "two can be as bad as one" if you forget Rippetoe's affirmative action. A good or great training buddy can help you move on up with accountability. A not-so-good buddy can bring you down.

Strength helps you age well, or to down age. (I strongly prefer the term down aging to anti-aging and super-aging.) Strength makes you a generational outlier on the "right" side of the bell curve for GenX performance and healthspan. This is the third time I assert that a great outlier like you performs on a par with someone *ten years younger*. This is your *downaged* advantage. I wager that you can take advantage of extras in that "saved" decade. Bump your kinetic count again.

THREE BODY PLANES

Formal names for your three axes of movement, or body planes, sound strange unless you are a trained kinesiologist. Simply, your muscles and joints move your body or limbs from 1.) front to back, 2.) side-to-side, or 3.) in twisting movements. Isn't that a *plainer* picture than sagittal, frontal, or transverse planes?

1. When you move from front to back, such as doing a hip hinge motion or a good-morning stretch, you are moving *sagitally*. Or when you carry weights in a farmer's walk. (You will gain familiarity with these and other motions in pages to come.) Or when you perform a forward or backward lunge maneuver or a push-up to improve your dynamic strength. Or hold a plank position for endured stability and strength. These important movements and stable positions work your sagittal body plane as shown in Figure 1.1.

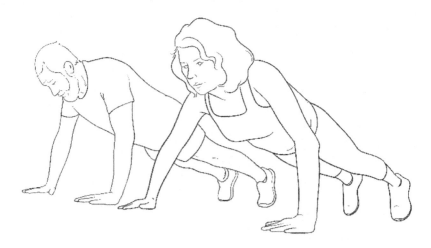

Figure 1.1: GenX Push-Up Planks in Sagittal Plane

2. When you move your body or torso or limbs in its side-to-side direction, you are working in your body's frontal plane. Envision and execute a side straddle hop (aka jumping jack), or a side lunge, and you are working your body in the frontal plane. If you're feeling young and frisky, a cartwheel is also executed in your frontal plane or axis.

3. When you twist your body or torso in a corkscrew-like motion, you are working in the transverse body plane as shown in Figure 1.2. Tee up and take a golf swing, make a discus throw or row in a "sweep" crew shell. As you execute these moves, you are doing great work in your transverse body plane. C'mon baby...

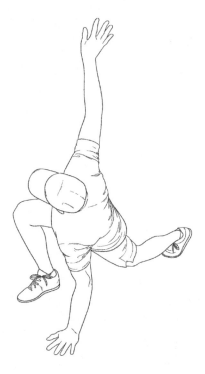

Figure 1.2: A Transverse Plane Twist in
World's Greatest Stretch (WGS)

DO THE LOCOMOTION

Now, put wonderful motions in all three of your axes or your three body planes in sequence. I suggest one *great* combination move to perform when you are ready for locomotion. Your functional strength, combined with stretching and stability, are used in this byzantine-sounding exercise, the Turkish Get Up. The origin of this maneuver may or may not be Turkish, yet its exotic name may entice you to give it a go. Make it your great GenX goal to move in all three body planes in every resistance workout and in your activities of daily life (ADL.)

THE TURKISH GET UP

When you execute a Turkish get up, or TGU, with a weight held consistently overhead, you are assuredly a strong, flexible, and stable GenX. TGUs challenge your strength, flexibility, and stability in all three body planes of motion. This three-pane image below (Figure 1.3) shows the starting position, midway position, and final standing position of a guy's weighted TGU while keeping the arm straight and weight (kettle bell) overhead.

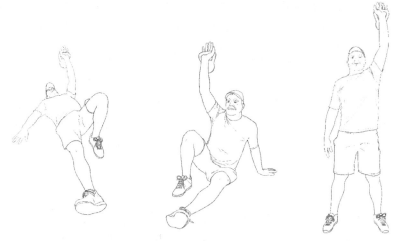

Figure 1.3 Three Turkish Get Up phases.

Ladies and Gentlemen:

- You will be truly **great** at Turkish get ups (TGU) by using a weighted object that *approaches* one-half of your bodyweight. That is strong stuff indeed.
  - o Ladies – can you carefully complete a TGU with a heavy weight or kettlebell?
  - o Gentlemen – how about you?
- Be assured that a TGU—at your bodyweight or with any external weight lifted—is very good motion as medicine.

THREE CHARACTERISTICS

Here is another trio of kinetic counts. You become *Strong to Save* by moving stuff with:

    a. volume,
    b. intensity, and
    c. tempo.

We professional trainers develop training principles to help each *individualized* client achieve characteristic gains. The *PPST3* by Mark Rippetoe that I mentioned earlier is one such a program guideline. Templates are also available from certifying organizations like the National Federation of Professional Trainers (NFPT). Many manuals or checklists for weightlifting and resistance training protocols / progressions are available online. In most PT guidelines, five training principles are common for an individual's procedures over time:

    1. Overload,
    2. Work specific muscle groups or regions,
    3. Avoid losing strength gains made to that point,
    4. Perform variable routines to keep the work interesting, and
    5. Achieve appropriate rest, restoration, and recovery.

Yes, you've already seen a passel of numbers and concepts to help you become a great GenX. Stay tuned as there are more to come in your fit map. You should remember, consider, and then tap into those training guidelines to reach and sustain your desired level of strength.

    ✓ You will move your bodyweight via lift, push, pull, twist, or carry movements.
    ✓ Or you will lift, push, pull, twist, and carry external weights or objects.

In either case or in both cases in a hybrid sense, It will be *your* individual package. A tailored package or plan that is designed with volume, intensity, and tempo variables for your weighty movements. For example, if it is your passion to build skeletal muscle size (hypertrophy) and strength for a muscle group or groups:

- You shall safely perform a total of twenty-four to thirty-six repetitions in two to three sets for an exercise or movement (volume).
- You will use a sufficiently heavy weight or resistance that your last repetition is difficult (intensity).
- And you will safely move that weigh in a slow range of motion for each repetition (tempo). A nominal five - to seven-second repetition provides a good time under tension (TuT) for your muscle groups in this hypertrophy and strength protocol.

Dwayne "the Rock" Johnson advocates, as I do, your particular attention to the negative or eccentric phase of a muscular movement. Trust him and me if you seek optimal gains. You'll soon gain a working knowledge of this eccentric phase of muscle movement.

Yes, it is perfectly fine to be a little bit *eccentric* when dealing with your ten-million-dollar physical bank.

THREE LEVELS OF STRENGTH AND FITNESS

Where are you now in this *triple tier* of strength levels?

1. General (decent) strength and fitness? Can you perform work or at about the same rate or activity measure(s) as your "peers by age and gender"? This fundamental level of strength fitness means that you can carry on your daily activities with about the median/average of strength and fitness level of your age and gender peers. Hence, my descriptor of "decent" isn't all bad, yet it *isn't* good or great. If you are consciously content

with this ordinary strength tier, then you may *concede* that achievable decade of health span savings. This is your personal choice. After all, it is *your* physical bank.

Remember that the difference between ordinary and extraordinary is that little bit extra. A higher level of strength via those invested extras may appeal to you as it did and does for me. You'll likely die harder and later. That is quite an extra.

2. Incremental (good) fitness and strength? You apply your time and talent in your journey to become stronger and fitter than *about* three-quarters (75 percent) of your age and gender peers. This is "pretty good" strength. Notice that my strength triad doesn't conform to "normal" bell curves in statistical senses. It is *not* intended to be normal. Remaining well past forty isn't "anything-but-normal strength and power" versus a general population. It is about you living better and probably longer because you forced your body to adapt to resistance loads you placed upon it. A good GenX takes sthenic strength to heart and deed. Stay tuned for functional strength measures as good goals if you want to be stronger than about three quarters of GenX of your age and sex.

3. If a competitive bent or a high achievement beckons, then a great third level of strength and fitness is calling you. I hope that greatness appeals to you and your physical banking!

Competitive (great) fitness and strength?! Your combination of natural abilities, plus commitment, developed strength, and power place you in the *top* 5–10 percent of all GenX athletes of your gender and calendar age. This heady tier for strength is a worthy goal with very worthy outcomes. Many of us can strive for and even achieve strength excellence. And, another drumroll, you are quite likely to enjoy that downaged decade of added health span. Another kinetic bump follows.

FOUR TYPES OF HUMAN STRENGTH

Please don't think too *deeply*. Just acknowledge that a DEEP mnemonic aid can help you plan a balanced journey to build and sustain "that on which all else is based":

1. **D**ynamic
2. **E**ndured
3. **E**xplosive
4. **P**eak.

Let's discuss 'em before you use 'em often ...

1. **Dynamic** strength is one's muscular power exerted in *repeated* motions. A notorious example was a workout of Supreme Court Justice Ruth Bader Ginsburg. Ladies and gentlemen, if that eighty-something cancer survivor could work on her dynamic strength, then "younger folks" should too. May your dynamic work please the court.

2. **Endured** work is your second category of human strength. Endured strength involves a lengthy set of resisted movement(s) to withstand one's bodily fatigue. Personal trainer David Chu offers this operational meaning for *endured strength*: "It's being able to do something that takes *significant strength for a very long time*. That's very different from, say, working toward a max(imum) single squat repetition."

A farmhand's fatiguing work during long harvesting days is certainly *endured* strength. Even if you're in an urban workout scene, a farmer's walk is a fine endured strength measure of gym age or fitness age for men and women. Gym age, you say. You betcha. Strive for the endured gym age or fitness age strength of *younger* people because you can. Let's consider another endured strength measure to get passionate about ...

One of the finest examples of GenX endured strength is to perform a single pull-up in a one-minute period. Yup, take thirty seconds to pull yourself up with your chin topping over a high bar. Then take thirty seconds in a very slow, negative (eccentric) motion to lower to your full "hung" position. This is an epitome of being *gym strong*. Ladies, I applaud recent acknowledgements that most of you *can* pursue pull-ups like gentlemen can. You may not complete as many repetitions, yet you are strong if you do them at all. Complete one pullup in an endured 30 seconds, and I consider you to be great.

Metabolic weight sessions are other examples of endured strength activities. The metabolic strength protocol is to constantly and slowly change your muscles' contracted or extended lengths in each exercise set. Try executing as few "reps" as possible in ninety to 120 seconds for a chosen exercise. Sound easy? I think you will find that is not the case.

Choose a medium weight and then perform a repetition in about fifteen seconds—*then* keep on keepin' on with more slow reps until your first timeout is reached. Then move quickly to your next planned exercise set without rest (nominally about ten seconds) and restart a next exercise. These "metabolic" regimens are short and efficient strength workouts. Plus, they are superbly effective too. Call or write me if you'd like to know more about these slowly executed endured strength series.

You'll please yourselves and me when you learn to love functional *endured* strength moves like the farmer's walk, or that full minute pull-up, or metabolic regimens. Your body, your spouse or significant other, and your grandkids will thank you for your endured strength. I could also add lower sick-care costs as a major beneficiary too.

3. **Explosive or elastic** strength is a force you exert *quickly over distance*. Did you see or hear about how high a former professional athlete, J. J. Watt, could box jump? His fifty-seven-inch box leap as a 280-pound football player was truly *explosive* or *elastic*. J. J. is what one might label a physical "freak of nature," so set your own non-freaky, mortal *plyometric* strength goals. Plyometric literally means "more measure." Plyometric strength operationally results from an activity that enables a muscle to reach maximal force in the shortest time possible. Folks

like J. J. Watt trigger their "fast twitch" muscle sequences elastically. The technical name for such a quick-draw muscle motion is a *stretch shortening cycle* or *SSC.* J. J. Watt has a very short SSC. I do *not.* Watch for short SSCs of women and men in Olympic power lifters. Watch elite CrossFit® competitions for both women and men too. Those outlier athletes are blessed with explosive strength and short SSC's. Perhaps you are too.

Our grandkids like the *Incredibles* movie characters, including an elastic-limbed mom. Her SSC is awesome. Granted, these *impulsive* powers and heavy lifts in blinks of the eye can't be humanly repeated as dynamic strength for longer periods of work. We're not transformers or incredible cyborgs, after all. Please take away this: you *can* strive to be the best that you can be for your own elasticity (SSC).

4. **Peak** strength is your generated maximum force, irrespective of time. The current world record deadlift is a "mere" 1,155 pounds (524kg) of dead weight. Lifting over half an English ton of stuff to one's waist level is one herculean load, which couldn't be accomplished without peak or absolute strength.

Note: Your starting load to progress toward peak strength could be a five-pound bag of flour or an overnighter suitcase, rather than a half-ton truck. Remember, you're not record holder Zydrunas Savickas or Captain America. Start with a dead weight that you can handle safely and then progress to heavier objects in your unique strength program as you adapt to imposed demands. Your specific adaptation to imposed demands means another entry in your growing glossary, namely S.A.I.D.

We also classify "hysterical" rescues as incidents of peak strength. We humans are fascinated by such Herculean hoists. For example: a special Samaritan, Tom Boyle, raised a Chevy Camaro high enough to save a person trapped underneath it, (under *very* special circumstances) as the BBC reported. Tom briefly overrode his body's safety circuitry with adrenal boosts in his peak lifesaving lift. By the way, Tom was a very big and very strong dude who was at the right place at the right time to be a momentary overriding hero. Should a great GenX work all four types of human strength? Yes.

Think and move like a cross-fitter, a pentathlete, or a decathlete or a competitive master's athlete who uses *multiple* types of strength on his or her journey.

Develop all four: dynamic, endured, elastic, and peak strengths.
Be X factor strong—in all four of these ways.

Lift on to sustain strengths in the spirit of J. J. Watt, Tom Boyle, and the *notorious* Ruth Bader Ginsburg. I advocate lifting to perform well and feel good, which you will. But wait, there is another nice perk.

Strength efforts define your body shape in pleasing aesthetic ways. Mirrors, kids, drunks, and Lululemon tights do *not* lie. None of these sources lie about your buff, downaged body. Repeat after me: It is all right to be both humble and appreciated. Go ahead. Kindle appreciative looks and ignite animal spirits. I add one spiritual foursome from a legendary guitarist, Carlos Santana. Santana is still going strong and performing at age 76 (in 2023). I share his four "D" X factors that shape his adult life:

1. Devotion.
2. Dedication.
3. Discipline.
4. Diet.

Santana recently told one reporter, "it has served me very, very well, because I look better than a lot of people my age and have a lot of brain cells firing!" Amen.

You may know that social saying that whenever and wherever four shall meet, they may be a *fifth*. Here we go...

FIVE WAYS TO MOVE HEAVY STUFF IN YOUR LIFE

Let's count those five resisted movements again: 1.) lift, 2.) push, 3.) pull, 4.) carry, and 5.) twist. These movements are *not* five easy pieces. Rather, they *are* quite hard handfuls and deservedly so. Each of these strength movements needs to be scheduled and performed for the rest of your great healthspan. Do the work, and don't stop 'til you get enough of each and all movements. Do not stop moving stuff unless you want to concede 7-10 extra healthy years. Conversely, go ahead and stop moving if you accept a *20 percent loss* of healthy years in your lifespan. As the respected Dr. Michael Joyner offers,

> "The idea is to live a long time and then die
> quickly with minimal disability."

Your strong to save constitution exemplifies Joyner's ideal of a long life and quick death.

Think of England's dearly departed Queen Elizabeth II as a model for Joyner's ideal. She was healthy as a walker and horseback rider. She was here today, but then she was quickly gone tomorrow at ninety-six years of age (in 2022). A long health span almost equaled her lifespan. That is truly what I am writing about. Repeat after me: Live longer, die harder and later.

One, two, three, four and five ... Now that you've read these five kinetic counts, I bet that you want to get started with a royal example. So, here you go with the king and queen of weightlifts, the deadweight lift or *deadlift* for short.

Whether or not you are new to regal resistance moves, the deadlift is one perfect move to get strong. By the way, one repetition is a very good number if you are demonstrating bodily peak power as suggested in Figure 1.4.

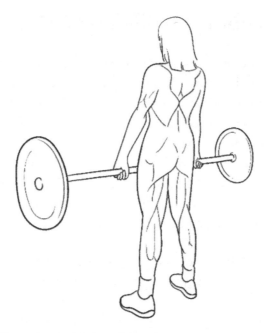

Figure 1.4: Lady's Deadlift at the Isometric (Top) Phase

Ladies and gentlemen: there is merit to our adage that being strong is the new skinny. Each deadlift works many major muscle groups of your body in the sagittal plane. You will adjust the volume, intensity, and tempo of your deadlifts in your unique progressions over time. As I S.A.I.D.—you will see results in eight to twelve weeks—trust me. Never neglect preplanned and executed variations of volume, intensity, and tempo for your progressive work and play. Never concede to weakness, never!

Remember those four D.E.E.P. types of functional strength? You do the math for those four strength variables to boost your health span and lifespan. Please make a note that lifting heavy stuff does challenge both your musculoskeletal system *and* cardiovascular system. Example: A great GenX deadlifter may experience a transient blood pressure that rises to a reading of 300/200mmHg in a peak lift. That is not a typographical error. That is a stress point reminder to gain medical approval for safe lifting. Now, take a deep, cleansing breath to be ready and set.

READY, SET

A set count for three categories of strength-building follows. A strength set is a preplanned number of repetitions for a movement or strength exercise. For example, a "straight" power set of deadweight lifts could be three to six repetitions before taking a rest.

Now, there are "advanced" types of resistance sets for great GenX folks. Great GenX lifters may encounter drop sets, super sets, compound sets, pyramid sets, or TuT sets. I encourage you to consider some of these specialized protocols as you progress on your journey. I know that you will be set.

General guidelines for safe deadlifts in three set categories follow. Note: other lifts conform to these set protocols too.

Endurance and Toning? Execute about fifteen or more safe deadlifts per set at slow tempo with light to medium resistance. Don't worry if you don't have ready access to an Olympic barbell. Find a heavy sandbag, suitcase, downed tree log, or an oversized tire or beer keg filled with your favorite IPA and safely lift away. Keep your rest intervals between endurance and toning sets fairly short.

Hypertrophy and Strength? Execute eight to twelve safe deadlifts per set at moderate tempo with heavy resistance. Your rest and recovery period is longer than it is for endurance and toning. Wait about ninety seconds between sets or use your recovering heart rate of about 120–130 beats per minute before you begin another set. Achieve a nominal twenty-four to thirty-six total repetitions per workout to gain hypertrophy and strength gains over time.

Power? Execute three to six safe deadlifts per set quickly with a *very* heavy resistance weight or load. Then take a relatively long time to recover before getting another royal grip to powerlift in the sagittal plane.

Note: New or relatively new weightlifters should work on their endurance and muscle-toning first, then move to hypertrophy and strength-building before powerlifting in planned progressions over time. Yet your successful journey doesn't need heavy metal.

Consider starting your own "big band" era for resistance work instead of heavy metal objects. A resistance band of a chosen deadlift "load" can be looped under your feet at shoulder width. Crouching as necessary, you can comfortably grip/grab the resistance band with both hands. Then perform a hip hinge to a low position with your head in a neutral position. Then, exhale as you lift upward against the band's resistance, possibly adding a shoulder shrug at the top of your deadlift. *Ta Da.*

I'm not writing about theory here. Like Mark Rippetoe, I'm sharing practical and functional strength options with you. The ever-young Tom Brady practically relied on resistance bands rather than metal dumbbells or barbells as he built a greatest of all time (GOAT) pro-football legacy. Adapt and excel, even if you don't succeed TB12 as the GOAT. And mix things up in your portfolio.

BORING, NOT

Yes, there are wonderful variations of your deadlifts to keep life interesting. Variations focus on specific muscle subgroups and bodily balance used in your complex "whole body" deadlifts. Three variants follow as examples to keep your royal resistance moves interesting:

1. Execute a single leg deadlift variant (Figure 1.5) with a kettle bell that adds unilateral stability to your dynamic or endured strength move.

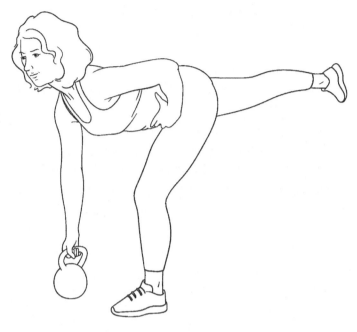

Figure 1.5: A GenX Lady's Single Leg Deadlift

The strong folks at MasterClass.com offer a complete "HOW TO" guide for this wonderful unilateral variant.[1]

2. How about a bilateral Straight Leg DeadLift (or SLDL)? Some lifters abbreviate this lift as a RDL for Romanian DeadLift. This variant to the "normal" or Olympic style DeadLift accentuates your hip hinge. What's more, the RDL unilaterally works your posterior chain of muscles, connective tissues, and bone.

    That's right. Your royal strength involves more tissues than just skeletal muscles. Your fascia, ligaments, tendons, cartilage, and bones are also present and accounted for.

3. And try Jefferson deadlifts. This is a normal or Olympic deadweight lift with one exception. You straddle the barbell for either a straight leg or traditional deadlift. In a Jeffersonian

way, you add asymmetry and anti-rotation features to your royal family of dead lift options.

There are more Deadlift options, like Sumo Deadlifts, whose positions you might imagine by the name. All deadlift variants shift imposed demands and reinforce your capabilities as a great GenX.

Should you perform safe deadweight lifts when you are medically cleared? I argue that the answer is yes. Compound exercises with loads that are heavy for you are quite clearly … tailored medicine.

Whatever deadlift variant becomes your favorite, try 'em all out so that you will maintain your enthusiasm and be a strong member of a chain gang.

CHAIN GANG

"Kinetic chains" are interrelated segments that produce your everyday actions to walk, run, jump, and lift. A kinetic chain is "the collective effort of two or more joints to produce movement," according to the National Strength and Conditioning Association (NSCA). You will leverage two types of kinetic chains to build and maintain your strength: (1) closed chain and (2) open chain movements.

I advocate your focus on closed-chain strength movements, though there are valid reasons to do "isolated" open chain strength moves too. As *Men's Health* magazine advises, open-chain exercises— like bicep curls and bench presses—focus on specific muscle groups or regions in relative isolation. Such isolated open-chain moves were responsible for the buff bodies in the beach football scene of *Top Gun: Maverick*. That is just an observation of mine.

But first things first, ladies and gentlemen … The royal lift you just "weighed," the dead(weight) lift, is a closed chain resistance move. Your feet for a regular deadlift (or a foot in a SLDL), stay(s) in fixed contact with the ground. Your hip and knee joints open and close in relation to the floor as a fixed position. Think of your "chained" ankles, knees, hips, and shoulder-joint movements in relation to the fixed floor. Voila – you gain compound interest in your physical banking efforts.

As you use multiple hinging and rotating joints, the dead(weight) lift is also known as a *compound* exercise. Life is a wonderful compound activity. Thus, compound lifts, rather than isolation lifts, should become a major part of your GenX strength regimen.

Think of those as compound interest generated in your physical banking efforts. One Time...

JUST ONE

Please dog-ear this performance benchmark once you commit to performing the king or queen of lifts.

✓ After proper dynamic warm-up, a beginner or novice lifter should be able grasp a loaded barbell, then lift *three-quarters of her or his bodyweight* from the ground to a knee-level with a final straight-back position. Three-quarters of a person's bodyweight as a starting lift is considered decent or good. Thus:

- A 140-pound lady should be able to deadlift 105 pounds for one safe repetition, known as a one repetition maximum or 1RM.
- A 180-pound gentleman should be able to deadlift 135 pounds for one safe repetition, known as a 1RM.

✓ Yes ... this starting 1RM benchmark of 75 percent of bodyweight is valid for both genders.

Why is the deadlift truly royal? The deadlift barbell loading is the heaviest of any weightlift that a human can perform.

Although the single deadlift world record for huge and jacked strongmen was over 500 kilograms in 2020 (1105 pounds), some smaller and (perhaps) more natural weightlifters in their middle-ages lift up to two to three times their bodyweights for a single repetition. Look up master's power lifting records for validation … Two recent records are:

1. A forty-something Danish female lifter, weighing 66 kilograms (Kg), or about 145 pounds, deadlifted (1RM) 233 Kg (514 lbs.) for a lift-to-bodyweight ratio of over 3:1.

2. A male Ecuadorian GenX powerlifter of 87 kilograms (191 lbs.) maxed his deadweight lift (1RM) at 285 Kg (628 lbs.). This lift-to-bodyweight ratio of over 3:1 is assuredly great strength.

Why is this deadlift known as a power lift? Without *too heavy* a physics lecture, please ponder the aspect of power for a deadlift. I stress what a powerful *machine* you can be. We know that there is a mathematical relationship among weight, time, and distance to calculate the power generated by a weightlifter. A Brit named James Watt studied these relationships in relation to horsepower. He calculated that 746 foot-pounds per second were the same as 1 horsepower (HP). Admirers of Watt named the standard value of 1 foot pound per second after him.

Assume that the Danish female cited above lifted that weighted barbell 2.25 feet from the ground to her upright position. And assume that she generated that lift in three-quarters of a second.

POWER = Weight times distance (aka "work") divided by time of the effort. So, in English, units of power for her strong deadlift example:

- 514 lb. x 2.25 feet divided by three-quarters of a second.

This single power lift is equivalent to two horsepower, or 1.5 kilowatts generated. Granted, this is peak power, rather than the sustained electrical power to microwave your healthy popcorn or to power your air fryer.

Now, consider this generated power example by a decent GenX male weightlifter:

A 90-kilogram (198 lbs. bodyweight) male, aged fifty, deadlifts his bodyweight a vertical distance of 2.5 feet in one second. This power generated isn't quite a "horse" of 746 foot-pounds per second.

✓ His "current" deadlift power is about 198 lb. x 2.5 feet divided by one second. That is 495-foot pounds per second, or two-thirds of a horsepower.

A reader might take a moment and say, *yes but*, "I'm not a power weightlifter" … *Yes, but* I ride my bicycle and do indoor rowing as part of my activities of daily life. I don't see how deadweight lifts help me. Let me help you see how.

FLEX ALERT #4:

Your peak power generation has a *direct* correlation to sustaining power for endurance strength sports like cycling and rowing. Measuring watts or joules or foot-pounds per second is very much a thing for great GenX athletes.

Power generation is key if dying harder and being *strong to save* appeals to you. You get my theme about lifelong strong habits, don't you? Think of the 1960s trendsetter of television fitness, Jack LaLanne. If you are too young to remember Jack LaLanne, ask your parents about him. I *don't* suggest that you should strive to duplicate LaLanne's legendary power exploits. Yet, I do want you to etch his epitaph in your muscle memory: "It is better to wear out than rust out."

Rust from inactivity is verboten for a strong GenX. It is verboten now, and for the rest of your health span.

✓ One credible research study validated that eighty-something aged men could still build dynamic and endured leg strength in twelve weeks of tailored resistance training.[2] I am confident that this study extends to ladies too.

Here is one more thought about the royal power of a deadlift (and its many neat variations). As our "carbon" utility bills prove, *power does not come free.* Your DEEP powers expend stored energy from four bodily sources:

1. Intra-muscle (about four hundred total grams of mitochondrial energy are stored in your skeletal muscles)
2. In blood (a person weighing 160 pounds has only *four grams* of glucose circulating in her or his bloodstream)
3. In Liver (about a hundred grams of glycogen), and eventually
4. Stored fat (your optimal long-term energy source) for you to generate watts, joules, or foot-pounds per second. *Or* impressively generate "X" horsepower without whinnying or pawing the ground.

Although your brain isn't a muscle, it is a major "burner" of dietary kilocalories (Kcal) each day and night. A *Neuroscience Trends* article states, "The brain accounts for 2 percent of the body weight, but it consumes 20 percent of glucose-derived energy making it the main consumer of glucose ..."[3] Feed your head, as Grace Slick sang, as you feed your amazing skeletal muscles. And breathe mindfully. Your brain needs glucose, oxygen, and rest to keep your head in the game of life and strength training. I hope I've come clean about this.

FLEX ALERT #5:

Both your body's energy system and brain benefit from your clean eating of both macronutrients and micronutrients plus clean drinking, aka hydration. As a contextual point, regular vigorous exercise consumes *only* 20-25% of your body's utility bill per day.

The majority of your utility bill is rung up when you are at rest or moving and not exercising. There is a loaded term, non-exercise activity thermogenesis (NEAT), that accounts for a big part of your total energy expenditures when you are not sleeping. My message is that a great GenX is not sedentary. Burn calories, baby, burn throughout each day on your journey.

One survival process that impacts your body's *utility bill* is catabolism (the breakdown of muscle protein) before tapping fat as your "last resort" energy source. That's right. Your body *may* catabolize skeletal muscle storages for energy-sourcing before *it* taps white fat. This, for example, can happen if you lift heavily in a fasted condition. Timing may not be everything. Yet good timing for moving and eating *is* important for your physical banking. Now it's time for a math check.

Check my abacus as I evaluate expended energy and work accomplished in a specified period of time. First, a horsepower-hour is equivalent to 641 dietary calories (Kcal) burned or the work generated in sixty minutes or 3,600 seconds. What is my power point?

The more power a GenX athlete generates and/or the longer she or he generates it, the *more* dietary calories are expended to fuel that exercise.

✓ A great GenX athlete should understand stored energy and power generation to shape strength and body composition outcomes.

What you eat and when you eat it can make you *either* heavier and stronger, or lighter and stronger. Yup. Does a great GenX choose lean muscle or soft white fat in her or his body composition? Hmmm.

Let's put this in "nutrient bar" terms to reinforce the energy equations of a strength workout. Imagine that a GenX athlete eats a typical "energy" or nutrient bar before her or his interval strength workout. That bar's carbohydrate content is ~ 40 grams of sugar (plus a bit of fiber).

a. How many calories of potential energy is available from that bar after thirty to forty-five minutes of gut absorption time? The answer is 160 Kcal from the sugar in the energy bar.

How does this boost affect the workout and body composition? It depends on factors like the timing of the snack, the calories expended in the strength exercise, plus a person's size and metabolic rate.

b. An intense twenty-minute interval workout may expend 14 Kcal a minute, or about 280 total Kcal, depending on body size and the relative intensity of the intervals.

c. Is the energy equation *net* positive or negative?

To close one number-crunching loop, this exercise session totals more than 1 horsepower-hour. Remember, no pawing of the ground is needed to underscore the impressive power generated. Yet remember that a small energy bar eaten after the workout may negate all dietary calories expended. Knowledge of your utility bill is important, whether you want to gain muscle, lose white fat poundage, or stay where you are.

IT DEPENDS

The energy bar's absorbed sugar *can* help to fuel muscles as an augment to your body's four energy sources mentioned earlier. Yet, the energy expended in the interval session may not result in a "net" energy deficit for weight loss. There *is* a post-exercise afterburner effect called EPOC (excess post-exercise oxygen consumption) that boosts an athlete's metabolism for a "healthy" period after an intense workout is done. This net energy equation is altered if the athlete drinks or eats too many calories *after* the workout.

✓ Remember your training goal when working your energy equation.

Are you shedding white fat? If so, it is best to forgo the energy bar(s). Are you building your sarcomeres? If so, the energy bar can help refuel your muscular mitochondria with macronutrients, both the sugars and proteins' essential amino acids. An important note is that an average energy bar's absorption level may be *only* 20 percent efficient. Thus, the 10 grams of protein on the bar's nutritional label may *only* become 2 grams of absorbed protein in your system. I emphasize that a great GenX must become a true student of all strength enablers.

FLEX ALERT #6:

It takes you and me *a lot* of exercise-induced sweat and exhaled water vapor to "heat" stored fat.

A calorie is defined as the amount of energy needed to heat 1 gram of water by one degree Celsius. Elite athletes or special warfare operators like Navy Seals may "burn" 7,000 or more dietary calories a day. There's a hot lot of heating goin' on for them! Shift your energies now...

If you look at a meal replacement bar or candy bar in an English commonwealth country, you may see a different label for energy— joules. A wee teaspoon of sugar—or 4 grams—is *68* kilojoules of energy. Think twice before adding simple sugars to food or eating bars that can cause insulin problems and trigger fat storage.

Alternatively, you can grasp what it takes to transform just a gram of stored fat to bodily power. That intense twenty-minute workout we just reviewed transforms about a maximum of 30 grams of stored fat. As a pound is equal to 453 grams, it may take the athlete *fifteen* similar sessions to shed those 453 fatty grams as one pound of stored energy. *Fifteen.* This expenditure does not fully account for EPOC or for individual differences of body size and vital tissue composition. Yet the message is clear. *It takes an appreciable volume and intensity of strong moves to shed even a single pound from stored fat.*

Did you know that an average marathon run for a person in your generation equates to just *one* pound of white fat lost for those 42 kilometers traveled? Okay, this fit map is not called Lean to Save. However, being strong and being lean are both life-saving attributes. A great GenX gets leaner and stronger to move heavy stuff, move others, look better, die harder.

Your metabolism is increased by a higher ratio of your vital tissue called skeletal muscle. More "high octane" muscle means that more dietary calories are needed to keep your internal combustion engine running. Make a note that it is okay to idle occasionally.

Isn't it nice to think that an occasional (80/20) idle or break from clean eating doesn't mean long-term weight gain? In fact, a once-weekly break from dietary discipline is good for your metabolism and constitution.

Testing on Station WIFM, one, two, three, four, five ... Make your kinetic chain gangs work so that your next years are your best years. Generate D.E.E.P. power and make best use of your body's stored energy sources. Adapt to imposed demands. Move your body in three body planes with lifts, pushes, pulls, twists, and carries. And remember to match your energy intake with your chosen desires and goal.

You now know that kinetics count heavily for your physical banking and health spans. Mark Rippetoe is both strong and right.

Are you ready to listen for that matchup on station WIFM? You can call WIFM and request that it play "I'm Free" by the Rolling Stones. As I shared, a great GenX must be astute. If you weren't careful with your request, the WIFM disc jockey might play "I'm Free" by The Who.

The moral of this closing story is:

You can't always get what you want...but if you try... you get what you need to down age.

TINA.

Why Get Stronger and WIFM?

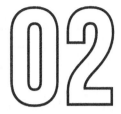

> "If you wish to know what man (or woman) will do, you must know ... desires and relative strengths."
>
> **—Bertrand Russell, Nobel Prize winner and oracle**

W hat a noble observation by a Nobel prize winner. Great and insightful GenX winners know where they are headed and do the work that needs to be done to get there. Even the great ones train like they are in second place.

What are *your* desires and *your* relative strengths? And how will you address those desires to improve your second-half-of-life strengths?

Now let's pound on what makes one particular group of winners special.

NORSEMEN

Question: Who is Thor's favorite pop star?
Answer: M. C. HAMMER.

You might have seen *The Vikings* series on a streaming service. Perhaps the hammering exploits of King Ragnar and his Norse folks kept you entertained and sane during COVID-19. If so, did you marvel at how that hardy group managed to row, raid, and revel even after some reached forty years of age? Keep those ardent voyagers in mind as you become strong to save.

Why must I get stronger, you may ask, or ponder WIFM? In no-nonsense Norse terms, Valhalla will have to wait a long time for those hardy souls with sthenic strength. Again, for emphasis, your down-aging strengths help you defer your visit to Valhalla by a decade. Your banked, *additional* decade of robust life and revelry is your WIFM. Period.

IMPECCABLE

Is it your desire to stave off or avoid illnesses and conditions that impact too many of your generational peers? Do you agree that it is OK to be lean and "cut"?

If so, tap others to help you stay *sterk* like Ragnar and his Viking cohorts. Stay *strang* like Braveheart, the Scottish highlander. Or stay modern-day strong like CrossFit champion Tia Claire Toomey. Trainers, workout buddies, and supportive life partners will help you make a strong progression. Find other strong links in your anchor chain.

Become a faultless student of your mind and bodily desires and strengths. Think and act like Epictetus, who still challenges each of us to this day, to "give an *impeccable performance.*" *As you read earlier, Epictetus was a physical disabled philosopher.* Why not transform into something superb for your own *impeccable* performances? Sagas of strength across time and distance are offered as your impeccable WIFM context.

WAY BACK

Strength was a matter of life and death in earlier eras. Three hundred Spartans who stalwartly faced Xerxes and his overwhelming force didn't become tough dudes without resistance training. Their strength training stimulated muscular adaptation to ready them for mortal combat. The underdog Spartan leader, Leonidas, is a hero of mine.

Yes, I am also a fan of Hercules and Samson. I also admire Stoics for their focus on time-efficient gymnasium workouts, and I am awed by Ulysses for *fortius* feats of his odyssey.

I do acknowledge that an imperfect Ulysses was delinquent, as he took a very long way home to Ithaca to reunite with Penelope after the Trojan Wars. Yet, that ten-year expedition gave us many samples of his strengths. He was both savvy and strong to avoid those sensual sirens, wasn't he?

Here is another way-back point. Another Stoic, Seneca, advised his followers to "give the body a workout without taking up too much time." In shorthand, *workout quick and often.*

Please dog-ear or highlight this Stoic's power point: There are *few* valid time-related excuses to skip weight training and resistance workouts. Three 45-minute workouts a week is about 1 percent(!) of your weekly time. Building your bank's ten-million-dollar cornerstone with only a 1-percent investment of time and talent is a very wise choice. Great gains, small investments... Even 5 minutes of daily strength, stability or stretching moves are beneficial.

You get strong, yet you invest far less workout time than it takes to get great in endurance exercises and activities.

That is a fact of human life, plus it is good news for your time-effective lifestyle, right? Note that I *am* chipping away at *"yes, but"* arguments that you cannot find time to get strong.

It takes many months or years to gain appreciable stamina. This is *not* true for gaining strength to save. As you read earlier, even elders in their eighties gained appreciable strength in three months of regular yet quick resistance sessions. Now that is an efficient feat. Right now, ladies?

FEMININE FEATS

Feats of strength were lauded in noble Olympic tradition, and through the years of history. Yet, feats of strength were not always manly. I offer this myth-buster that champions physical feats of Scythian women who were erroneously labeled Amazon warriors. A credible 2014 *National Geographic* article offers that: "Archaeology shows that these fierce women also smoked pot, got tattoos, killed—and loved—men."[4]

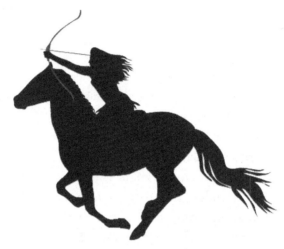

Figure 2.1: An Scythian Archer

No, those lady warriors did not have breasts removed to become better archers. No, they didn't come from Lesbos or from the Amazon region. Yes, they adapted to horse riding in ancient Scythia. And yes, their strong skills and prowess scared the bejabbers out of many Mediterranean males. Those *real* Amazons learned how to die hard at the expense of others. Ladies, why not embody the physical and mental spirits of those great Scythians? Be the strong equal of men.

Ladies, **do not** give in to "*yes but*" excuses like these lesser souls who *under*-invest in their bodies and banks:

- Social
- Psychological
- Lack of knowledge
- Lack of facilities or motivating coach
- Shortness of time.

Do or do not. Find ways or make them. Invest.

Today's great athletes (of both genders) present and "carry themselves" as did Braveheart, Ulysses, Stoics, and the Scythian females in days of yore. Aesthetic bodies are both hard and hard to overlook, aren't they? Reflect on this timeless wisdom of Socrates:

"It is a shame ... to grow old without seeing the beauty and strength of which (a) body is capable." Thank you, Socrates!

Who among us looks away from heavenly bodies?

ALLURING MUSCLE GROUPS

Seven magnificent muscle groups and body areas can draw attention and looks of envy or admiration:

1. Your "lats" or *latissimus dorsi*.
2. Your chiseled or visible abdominal muscles, officially called *rectus abdominus*.
3. An impressive neck that *no one* can call a "pencil neck."
4. Blacksmith forearms that suggest your grip is strong.
5. Distal deltoids (or *boulder shoulders*).
6. Your shaped gluteal muscles.
7. Your chest and shoulder girdle.

Your $64,000 question (before inflation) is: "how do I develop beauty and strength?"

YOU KNOW IT DON'T COME EASY.

Ringo Starr's lyrics tell us how. For both strength and sex appeal, you need to commit to *more than* weekend warrior recreation. Today's strong GenX athletes move stuff three times each week, a la Dwayne Johnson, or like Thor's action hero, M.C. Hammer's. Yes, use your setbacks to fuel progress, as GenX champ Dara Torres did. It definitely don't come easy for Todd Vogt!

Let me lob a geroscience[5] gem to reinforce the answer to that $64,000 question. Exercise is one profound and natural way to slow down your biological aging. Lovely.

ISN'T IT LOVELY?

So, Howard Stern doesn't host a show on station WIFM. Listen instead with passion for your personal DJ on WIFM. Passion fuels success in many endeavors.

You should get stronger to *down age* as your *geroscience* gain (where *gero* means aging). Say what? We know from recent and highly credible research that "right" exercises like interval training can extend your years of health while compressing those potential years of sickness. Again citing the respected Michael Joyner, MD, labeled this worthy odyssey as,

"the idea is to live a long time and then die quickly with minimal disability."[6]

Amen. Your station DJ is sharing what's in it for you: *Saving Strength*. Strength doesn't mean that you will be a muscle-bound meathead. Neither does strength mean that you must have boulders as shoulders, although defined deltoids do provide second looks in your direction. Rather, you have functional strength to fully work your kinetic chains (muscles, connective tissues, and joints) without injury. Strength means that others can and will depend on you.

STRENGTH IS THAT ON WHICH ALL OTHER IS BASED.

Note that pumping iron is not the sole or exclusive way to build and sustain your great strength. Nonferrous options for moving stuff include total resistance exercise (TRX) kits, resistance bands, surplus road tires, park benches, rucking backpacks, lumber, sandbags, ropes, or intimate partners.

You may have viewed how TV's Ninja warriors lift, push and pull, twist, and carry themselves past, around, over and through obstacles with nary a barbell in sight.

CrossFit athletes pursue many Workout(s) of the Day (WOD) that do *not* require barbells or kettlebells. The popular and arduous MURPH bodyweight workout is notably undertaken by many on Memorial Day to honor Michael Patrick Murphy. If you don't recognize this hero's name, use Doctor Google to look up his valor in *Lone Survivor.*

Another bodyweight example is a handstand push-up. Another is a unilateral pistol squat. Please give me a jingle if you can knock out a set of Handstand Push-ups, full Pistol Squats or do that one lone pull-up in an endured sixty seconds. I want to shake your hand with that very strong grip!

And for your road warriors and travelers, Station WIFM offers this Hotel Room workout of the day, or WOD:

twenty rounds of: five push-ups, five sit-ups, and five air squats *without* rest.

By now, you should be set on the value of strength training and know that there is almost always a way to find time to push, pull, lift, twist with, or carry. Sure, external weight or resistance is good. Bodyweight motion to sweat is just fine for periodic stints and when your workout box is a hotel room. Now, take a quick station break for this relevant seventies' song.

LET'S GET PHYSICAL

With sad tribute to the recently departed (2022) singer Olivia Newton-John, you should get physical, physical. Why not *let your body talk?* Your six training principles to get physical in strong and sexy ways are:

1. SPECIFICITY

Your dedicated resistance training efforts will (in eight to twelve weeks) improve muscles groups that are targeted, engaged, and challenged. You can and should pursue *specific* movements and workouts that achieve strong goals you established.

2. OVERLOAD

Get excited about working (aka loading) your amazing body. Choose progressions of volume, intensity, and tempo of repetitions to adapt to and tackle your imposed demands. I am not eccentric by personality. Yet I encourage *eccentric* focus just like Dwayne Johnson does. "Eccentric (negative) muscle contractions support the weight of the body against gravity and to absorb shock or to store elastic recoil energy in preparation for concentric (or accelerating) contractions."[7]

This is a great point in your fit map to address exercise- induced sweat and delayed onset of muscle soreness (DOMS). I love to endorse your sweaty work that helps you lengthen your health span. Sweat and soreness are your *no-kidding* sidekicks for strong successes.

With specific focus, and prudent overloading, you will sweat and trigger "right" cytokine flows. These little *cytokines* or *myokine* scouts (i.e., proteins within your immune system) biochemically sense your exercise stressors. Then they alert your feed-and-restore systems to cycle muscle recovery and growth. Note that these cytokine signals sense and respond to *inflammation*. Right!

You want *controlled* muscular inflammation, and you need *controlled* muscular inflammation. My cautionary caveat is this: you must give yourself adequate rest and anti-inflammatory sustenance to make your muscle fibers thicker and longer.

3. PROGRESSION

Speaking of progressions, you will apply types of *periodizations* that specifically overload your chosen kinetic chains to make gains in one or more chosen D.E.E.P. strength criteria. Did you dog-ear or highlight the D.E.E.P. descriptions of Strength in chapter 1's kinetic counts?

4. REVERSIBILITY

This is your use 'em or lose 'em principle of strength training. Lift, push, pull, twist, and carry stuff for the rest of your down-aged days. Or else...

FLEX ALERT #7:

It only takes about *two* weeks of inactivity, such as a fortnight's rehabilitation period, to relapse and lose some of your previous strength gains.

Think of a lower leg cast that is applied after a severe sprain or broken bone. Then imagine how quickly that casted calf or leg's circumference will lessen. Oy. 'Tis sad yet true that you and I fall from strength levels quicker than we can gain them. It takes eight to twelve weeks to gain strength versus two weeks to concede some of your gains. Stay strong to save.

5. BE F.I.T.T.

This four-factor F.I.T.T. mnemonic will help you stay principled and fit. F.I.T.T. is a shortcut for four specific strength factors, namely: 1.) Frequency, 2.)Intensity, 3.)Time, and 4.)Type. Note: This is a slight variation of the Volume, Intensity and Tempo triad for training that you read about in your **Kinetic Counts** chapter. Type is the variable added for you to be F.I.T.T. Here are more details for this "quad:"

Frequency: How often should you and will you perform your targeted exercise or physical activity?

Many athletes in GenX can recover from their exercise-induced muscle soreness (DOMS) to complete their full body* strength regimens three times a week with a day's rest in between sessions. In most cases, bodily recovery is completed with 36-48 hours between full body workouts. One normal schedule would be Monday, Wednesday, and Friday full workouts with each Sunday as a stretch day for full recovery. Alternately, one could do resistances sessions on Tuesday, Thursday, and Saturday while using Monday as the weekly day of rest and recovery.

*Full body workouts can be split into "halves" or components if dedicated athletes want to lift every day. Monday could be leg day, then Tuesday could be arm day and so on. When life happens and a day is missed, stress-not and resume a successful lifting habit that works for you.

Others, particularly as they age, may need two days of recovery between strength sessions (which equates to two strength workouts a week, every week. This could be a Monday-Thursday or Tuesday-Friday regimen for full body strength workouts.)

Now, light bodyweight exercises can be done every day without a major worry of muscle overload or DOMS. Note that I encourage every athlete to invest in a recovery day every week in your periodization. Low intensity stamina spins, and perhaps a wee bit of bodyweight motion and stretching are invaluable for these precious off days each week. Take note that proper recovery is essential to stay motivated and fresh. Reminder...

✓ Your main strength workouts should generate healthy exercise induced sweat and cause DOMS.

If you do *not* generate both positive factors, you should adapt and add more intensity or more exercise sets in extra time.

Intensity: Learn to assess your level of intensity during your physical activity via several of these indicators:

1. Training heart rate and recovery rate,
2. Measured power output (if available on an exercise apparatus),
3. Your relative perceived exertion (RPE),
4. Level and duration of bodily and mental fatigue, or
5. Your subjective score of Metabolic Equivalents (MET).[8]

Be fully aware of strength training at proper and safe intensities to benefit both your neuromuscular and cardio-respiratory systems. Self-awareness fits both leisure ADLs and more vigorous activities or exercise. Have you *"met"* a common subjective scale for exercise intensity or tolerance based on your oxygen consumption?

One Metabolic Equivalent of a Task (or MET) is scored as the resting oxygen cost while sitting and reading a book or while you are sleeping. From a physiological point, one MET is the product of oxygen consumption and time divided by your bodyweight in kilograms. Follow my arithmetic for this MET formula:

1 MET = 3.5 ml O_2 per kg body weight x minutes.

A tally of METs is offered in Table 2.1:

"The MET concept provides a convenient method to describe the functional capacity or exercise tolerance of an individual ..."[9]

Table 2.1 MET Levels versus perceived Exertion (source NFPT)

Describe your Exertion	MET Level(s)
At Rest or Light (Leisure) Activity Sleeping is 1 MET	1-4
Moderate Activity	5-8
Somewhat hard	9-14
Hard	15-16
Very hard	17-18
Extremely Hard	19-20

MET minutes combine intensity of one's energy expenditure with the next F.I.T.T. factor of Time. I bet that you are already thinking about a combined performance measure.

Combine frequency, intensity, and time for MET minutes. As a calibration point, Family Physicians and fitness professionals hope that you will work 450 to 750 MET minutes each week. By our Strong to Save standards, this is a *bare minimum* to improve healthspan. A great GenX works longer and harder than this average performance benchmark of 450-750 MET minutes per week.

As a great GenX, you commit to appreciable minutes of light to moderate exertion to build your endured capacity. Plus, you seriously commit a minority percentage of your workout time to hard work for your MET minute tallies. Show and Tell...

A Great Example: A Crossfit athlete invests 300 minutes each week in low intensity actions (moderate MET estimate of 7) to build capacity. That great GenX also invests in three strength sessions of 45 minutes each week (MET level estimate of 15).

✓ This GenX invests (300x7) +(3x45x15) = 4125 MET Minutes per week.

You can see how a great GenX invests frequently in time and effort to fortify that physical bank for healthspan.

Time: Time logically means the duration of your session and cumulative physical activity or exercise in each period. Remember that exercise-induced sweat takes time to generate. And never forget that it takes time, nutrients, and rest to build up what you "tore."

Suggestion: Keep your invested MET Minutes in a simple journal to monitor fitness trends and banked F.I.T.T factors.

Type: This final attribute in your F.I.T.T. kit classifies your chosen activity of daily life (ADL) or exercise. Some regimens can be demanding (with high power output, high HR, and higher METs), like CrossFit, boxing, singles tennis, distance bicycling, and wood chopping. Other activity types like walking and yard work can also lead to longevity, as validated in outlier communities called Blue Zones with many centenarians. Loma Linda California is one of those Blue Zones. If you are curious about Blue Zone lifestyles for longevity, research Dan Buettner at bluezones.com. After all, motion is medicine; and moving heavy stuff is very good medicine. One more time, let's consider what separates you from others in GenX with a sixth and final criterion.

6. INDIVIDUAL DIFFERENCES

Yes, you *are* an athlete. And yes, you are uniquely different in your capacities and capabilities. What works for Jill may not work for Jane. Successful habits for Bill may not work as well for Bob. Bespoke or tuned strength programs will produce better results than "cookie cutter" programs, I assure you.

These six factors are your physical bank principles for good reason. How these important principles apply individually to you is a key investment matter. Please reach out to me if you have questions. Or ask your personal trainer to help define your unique periodization to overload you, avoid reversibility, and stay "F.I.T.T. safely and specifically."[10] You are *not* just any *body*.

WHAT IS MY BODY TYPE?

As you drill into resistance regimens and delve into supporting lifestyle diets, make sure that you know your body type. You'll learn why this is important after you gauge which type you are.

Subjective body types, or somatotypes,[11] are partially genetic in their result. These physical classifications *guesstimate* your skeletal frame (bone structure and density) and body composition (of skeletal muscle and fat mass). Three body types (depicted in Figure 2.2) are:

1. **Ectomorph:** This body type is relatively thin, tall, and lanky. Ectomorphs may have trouble packing on vital skeletal muscle mass and fat. Imagine a marathon runner.

2. **Mesomorph**: This middle body type is likely to have a sturdy build, a bone structure with wider hips, thicker limbs, and more barrel-shaped rib cage than does an ectomorph. Ladies and gentlemen in this body type can intentionally or unintentionally put on weight. Yet they are also able to reduce their fatty weight. Think of a football tight end and a lady CrossFit athlete as examples.

3. **Endomorph:** If individuals find it tough to shed fat, they are probably endomorphs. They also tend to gain more (unhealthy) weight faster than mesomorphs and certainly ectomorphs. They may have a lower ratio of skeletal muscle mass in their physical classification than do mesomorphs. Endomorphs usually look broader when an observer views their frontal or posterior profiles. Think of an unfortunate obese person on the TV show *America's Biggest Losers*. Note: This body type can still have great GenX strength, as does a Sumo wrestler.

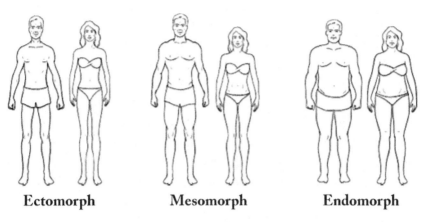

| Ectomorph | Mesomorph | Endomorph |

Figure 2.2 Three Body Types

Some of you may know the original intent of somatotyping someone was to link physical shape or physique with that mind's psyche and personality. A psychologist named W. H. Sheldon asserted this linkage in 1940. This psychological linkage is now discredited. Yet, body types, these three somatotypes, *do* matter when you consider strength-building and maintenance.

SIZE DOES MATTER

A female or male ectomorph may be *disadvantaged* if hypertrophy (building muscular size) is a strength goal. Note that I wrote *disadvantaged*, rather than "it's not gonna happen." There are many true stories about slim urban legends or "ninety-eight-pound skinnies" becoming big and strong. Jack LaLanne attributed his fitness and his successful career to youthful days as a scrawny kid who was bullied. Sexercise™ creator, Jason Rosell, does likewise. You'll officially meet Jason in chapter 6. Stay tuned.

As you'll read again and again for good reason, you are a unique GenX athlete. Thus, the physical training principles of specificity and overload come to play if a ninety-eight pounder wants to recruit then build brawny shoulders, bigger gluteal muscles, and strong legs for functional and/or aesthetic reasons. As a pleasurable sidenote, lithe ectomorphs may be very good indeed at the anaconda or other supple Sexercise movements you'll examine in chapter 6.

If an ectomorph wants to gain longer and wider sarcomeres, she or he should carve out a program of three full-body training sessions per week that highlight heavy, compound movements against resistance. And they will need to gain a surplus of macronutrients in their dietary lifestyles to get bigger over a several-month period. Note that half of skeletal muscle weight is water. So, hydration with filtered water is also important for your gain in muscle volume and mass from clean eating.

FLEX ALERT #8:

Ingesting about a gram of complete protein (that is, with all nine essential amino acids) per pound of body weight each day is a benchmark for muscle growth or hypertrophy over time.

So, a female GenX who weighs 144 pounds and who wants to offset sarcopenia should ingest up to 144 grams of complete proteins every day. A 200-pound male GenX should ingest up to 200 grams of complete protein daily if he is serious about maintaining or building his muscle mass. You'll read more about supportive diets in Chapter 8, "Your X Factors." There is more than a gram of truth in the adage that the route to strong and "cut" abdominal muscles is through your refrigerator door. Did you note that this rather daunting goal of daily protein intake is the same for both genders?

FLEX ALERT #9:

Folks of all three body types should celebrate tiny (i.e., micro) essentials and remember that some molecules are indispensable. Celebrate key indispensables with the mnemonic aid PVT. TIM HiLL. This acronym represents our nine essential amino acids: **p**henylalanine, valine, **t**hreonine, **t**ryptophan, **i**soleucine, **m**ethionine, **h**istidine[12], **l**eucine, and **l**ysine.

You are correct that there are ten, not nine letters in this acronym. Why? The *"i"* in *HiLL* is a convenient placeholder. As a minor point, there are new research studies that hint that histidine may be developed in our bodies. Mox nix, whether the number eight or nine is ground truth for a human's essential amino acids. A young biochemist with time on his hands came up with another mnemonic aid for those same nine essential amino acids:

"I Love Lucy Very Much, Please Try To Help."

Pick and choose one or devise your own memory aid if you are clever. The key is that you will not rebuild muscular microtears caused by training if you do not replenish your body with essential amino acids. Essential means that you must ingest and absorb these molecules from your food and drink, as your body doesn't generate them.

Now, circle back to the desirous quote for this chapter and to Epictetus the stoic's impeccable descriptor. What reflected image do you figure to see in your mirror? Why do I ask about figures?

A GenX with just ordinary or "decent" fitness probably has a higher, unhealthier waist-to-hip ratio (WHR) than a GenX who is good or great in fitness or gym years.

✓ A leaner waist and larger powerful glutes generally mean a longer lifespan and health span for a great GenX.

IT FIGURES.

A big waist can waste one's health span years and make that soul appear less attractive to most lookers. Plump Rubenesque bods are so antediluvian. "Cut" abdominals and strong glutes are two of your magnificent seven muscle groups that others view or imagine with pleasure or passion. Now, back to my main point about health span figures.

With a big waistline, you stand first in line to unbuckle unhealthy conditions called metabolic syndrome (MetS) and nonalcoholic fatty liver disease (NAFLD). These two conditions can waste one's health span and lifespan. What a preventable shame.

So, pursue and maintain a lean waist with strength training and lifestyle habits of diet and rest as enablers.

- Ladies, this means that your waists should be less than thirty-two inches (circumference) to be rated as *low* risk for cardiovascular disease (CVD).
- Gentlemen, if your waist at its narrowest circumference is less than 37 inches, you are statistically at *lower* risk for CVD.

What was the number-one killer of American adults in 2022? CVD!

Please bear in mind that somatotypes are generalized body classifications, so folks may not be cookie-cut to a particular class. Your fit map author puts more faith in measurements like body fat percentages and waist-to-hip ratios than generalized body profiles. How do you measure up?

MEASURE FOR MEASURE

A health professional may have calculated your body-mass index (BMI) at some point. This *outdated* statistical measure was suited for young, white males, European conscripts in the early nineteenth century, as calculated by a well-intentioned Doctor Adolphe Quetelet. Do you see anything missing from this statistical approach? Hint: *Women are missing.* Hint: *Modern macronutrient-rich diets too.* Hint: *Other ethnic types and professions that can affect one's height and weight are also lacking.*

FLEX ALERT #10:

Waist to Hip Ratios are *far better* measures to gauge your prospects for both lifespan and health span than outdated surrogate BMIs.

Your calculated BMI is simply unfit for many in GenX (and for folks in other generations too). BMI *does not* accurately measure lean tissues in its rubric. Thus, athletes of both sexes get misclassified as being overweight or obese when they have *actual* low body-fat measures. Anecdotally, one all-world NFL receiver, Jerry Rice, was classified by a doctor as obese by the BMI estimation. Anyone who has seen Jerry Rice knows that his low body fat, sleek muscles, and tall frame are anything but obese!

I am so adamant about shortfalls of BMI measures that I offer this extended quote from one of my professional articles:

"To give credit where credit was due, Dr. Alfonso Quetelet was an amazing nineteenth-century statistician. His Quetelet Index for "the average man" was rephrased as "Body Mass Index or BMI" by scientist Ancel Keys in 1972. Health professionals now recognize that a male's tendency to store dangerous white and visceral fat around his middle (waist) better marks mortality risk than is a standalone 'surrogate' index like BMI."[13]

A male's high weight or body mass doesn't necessarily mean he's unhealthy or suggest CVD risk factors. However, males with waist measurements of thirty-seven inches or more are truly at high risk for CVD and possibly some diet-influenced cancers. To be redundant, the high-risk measure for ladies' waist measures start at thirty-two inches.

A very effective way to assess health risks is to look at a full-length mirror (with your shirt or blouse removed). One can—and should—use a simple two-part measure to gauge sightings of mortal danger. Find a $3.00 cloth tape measure to get this done.

1. First, measure your waist—half-way between your hip (iliac) crest and lower rib cage. Record that current measure.
2. Then measure the widest circumference of your hips.

With this second measure as denominator, calculate your measured waist (numerator) over hip ratio (denominator)—or WHR.

Guys: If your current waist measurement is bigger than your hip circumference, you are at high risk for *your* top killer: atherosclerosis cardiovascular disease (ASCVD). Ditto for ladies when a waist measurement approaches hip circumference. Remember that ladies also have ASCVD as a leading cause of death. Detailed steps in lifestyle and diet that improve WHRs are a weighty topic beyond the abridged intent of your fit map. Let us stay at a summary level and consider three factors that lower WHRs:

1. Change your energy equation. Plan and execute timed exercise and diet to deliberately shed central obesity and lower waist circumference.
   o Intermittent fasting is one method to challenge your energy equation to get leaner.
2. Hypertrophy. Plan and execute gluteal and hip exercises to add muscular circumference to hips.
3. Tighten your natural corset. Regularly tone and tighten your bodily midsections with deep core exercises for:
   - Trans versus abdominus (TVA)
   - Internal obliques (IO)
   - Psoas muscles.

Ladies, WHR works for you like it does for gentlemen, so please note that I'm always thinking about you too. Your healthy WHR measurement is comparatively lower than for a man, even if you are not Barbie. That's the way life is, and viva la difference!

Dog-ear this unfailing tenet please:

✓ A GenX of either gender with a lean waist and with powerful glutes is healthier, fitter, and will probably live longer.

That is inarguably the *shape* of things. Hips and belly fat do not lie.

The World Health Organization (WHO),[14] stresses that *healthy* WHRs are:

- 0.9 or less in men
- 0.85 or less for women.

In both men and women, a WHR of 1.0 or higher *increases* the risk for heart disease and other conditions. Yes! Resistance training, particularly when you incorporate interval-like sessions, assuredly helps you get leaner and healthier by changing this health span and lifespan figure. Remember, just like Shakira's hips, that waist-to-hip ratio *doesn't* lie. And that's the truth.

TRUTH OR DARE

People who carry more weight around their midsections (imagine an apple-shaped body profile) are at higher risk for ASCVD and diabetes than are those who carry more weight in their hips and thighs (as a pear-shaped body).[15] Death wishers—pad your midsection with white fat and Saint Peter will see you sooner. Down-agers—you can say *hasta luego* to the pearly gate keeper. For you, Valhalla will have to wait. Wait for about ten years.

SO, WHAT TO DO ABOUT IT?

Here's the simple-yet-hard action step: Make motion your medicine and progressively move heavier stuff that stands in your way. Dwayne "the Rock" Johnson appreciates that action. With an intensity principle of strength training in your mind, get your left ventricle a-pumpin'. As you register your exercise-induced sweat, many good things happen. You can burn more calories (dietary kilocalories) than you choose to ingest. Sweat more, eat a bit less, period. No tricks, and space out your sweet treats. You can lower your non-exercise stress levels. You can sleep better, and better sleep together.

There are *not* many downsides to these physical banking outcomes, are there? Yes, you can and should experience DOMS, that delayed onset of muscle soreness after workouts. Celebrate muscular soreness. Now, if joint are discomforted or painful, then that is another matter. But exercise-induced muscle soreness is to be achieved and applauded. Back to those dietary calories and energy equation. Calories *do* have a lot to do with aesthetic and strong body compositions.

We have more, way more calories stored as fat than we have available as carbohydrates (or muscle) to power our sustained activities. This is important, as some of us are natural "fat burners" or lean ectomorphs who have metabolic "burn" ratings to stay lean, as compared to mesomorphs and endomorphs who do not. We need healthy fats for many bodily functions. Fat is an awesome energy source, as each gram of fat provides nine dietary calories (Kcal) of energy. Healthy fats and fatty acids from olive oils, nuts, and avocados are both necessary and energizing when used in moderation.

Many of us are *not* natural fat-burning ectomorphs, and it's not our fault for being mesomorphs or pudgy endomorphs. It is possible to be a great GenX if any of these 3 somatotypes. Yet it is also your mandate to get as lean as possible for as long as humanly possible. Lean and Learn.

LEAN

Lean is a four-letter word. It is a fine four-letter word and acronym when health span and lifespan are your dependent variables. Here's how you and I should LEAN:

> L—lighten
> E—enhance
> A—activate
> N—nurture.

Whatever your natural body type (or somatotype), being leaner is a true, achievable, and eye-pleasing virtue. Strive to become leaner on your sustained journey with clean eating. Why? Central obesity causes bodily inflammation. And leaner folks tend to be more vital in their activities of daily life (ADL). Eat cleaner and add quality strength training so that you can achieve LEAN. I *didn't* say that this achievement was easy. Still, I mentioned that an added *decade* on this crazy planet was a viable goal. Yes, your mesomorphic author strives for this down aging result. And yes, you should too.

OK, SO WHAT CAUSES THIS ENDOMORPHIC SHAPE?

Genes are one root cause. Stress is another factor behind it. When facing episodic or chronic stress, a body's adrenal system releases hormones including one called cortisol, "a steroid hormone, ...that regulates carbohydrate metabolism, maintains blood pressure, and is released in response to stress."[16]

In my terms, cortisol *adversely* impacts both protein synthesis and our normal responses to inflammation and immunity. Cortisol is also related to weight gain as it hampers insulin sensitivity. Our bodily cortisol secretions from chronic (extended) distress can lead to bad effects like these:

- A rise in blood sugar and blood pressure
- Lessened immune system resistance to infections
- Early cell aging.

Chronic stress equals early aging, a shorter life, and it eclipses one's chances to party hearty through your full second half. Know how cortisol rises, then whip it good with feel good hormone levels of serotonin, dopamine, and oxytocin. Once again, strength training helps to counter the ill-effects of cortisol (with sleep and clean lifestyle diets.)

Remember that you need to be in the correct mindset to achieve your physical banking goals. Stress does *not* help you except in danger zones. Perking up serotonin, dopamine, and oxytocin (aka the hugging hormone) *does* help your vitality.

Jerred Moon offers these 16 pearls to help you harness your cornerstone strengths and positive mindset[17] to get strong.

1. You are not Superman.
2. Take your time; learn slowly and correctly.
3. No perfectly ready person succeeds in a workout.
4. Focus! You are as ready as you will ever be.
5. The person with the fanciest clothes and equipment proves he or she has money, that's it.
6. If you are short of breath, you're working out.
7. When you're convinced you are about to lose or that you can't perform, you're right.
8. The important things are simple.
9. The simple things are sometimes very hard.
10. No plan survives the first contact intact.
11. If it's stupid but it works, it's not stupid.
12. If your workout is going really well, you aren't trying hard enough.
13. That "energy reserve" you plan to use later is now.
14. The only thing that is truly controlled in a workout is yourself.
15. The easy way generally means no results.
16. Working out is cheap; your life isn't.

Keep these sixteen mind games from Jerrod Moon in mind. Then form successful, impeccable habits to chill out and move stuff because your life isn't cheap.

WHAT IF I DON'T?

I will sound like an irritating broken record track if you *don't* form those strong habits. If you do not commit to strength, then your health span and lifespan may *drop* by about a decade. Period. That is about 3,650.25 healthy or total days that you will concede. Do you have interest in how your world turns? If you don't care, then you will experience "normal" onsets of sarcopenia and senescence. Then you might get to those pearly gates earlier than you might.

"The interest about sarcopenia, the age-related loss of skeletal muscle mass and function, is growing considerably. In 1989, Rosenberg proposed the term *sarcopenia* (Greek *sarx* or flesh and *penia* or loss) to describe this age-related decrease of muscle mass."[18]

Sarcopenia, or skeletal muscle atrophy (Figure 2.3) is caused by an imbalance between your sense-and-respond signals for muscle cell growth and teardown. Cell growth processes are "anabolic," while cell teardown processes that atrophy sarcomeres are "catabolic."

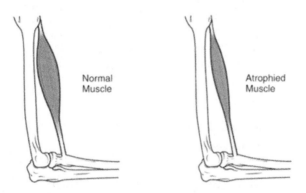

Figure 2.3 Normal and Atrophied Upper Arms (NFPT)

A lack of physical activity can result in muscle atrophy and serves as a key factor for sarcopenia. Atrophied muscles, ... are caused by nonactivity, illness, poor nutrition, and old age.[19] That is calendar aging – *not* fitness or gym downaging.

As you can see in Figure 2.3, the normal muscle on the left side is notably bigger than the atrophied biceps muscle group on the right side. Size matters for your second-half performance as a great GenX.

REDUX, WHAT'S IN IT FOR ME?

Your WIFM imperative, your *raison d'être* is that you will be a vital second-half performer for up to fifty years. Fifty years! You will be a great downaged outlier on the right side of the GenX bell curve. Let others be average or worse. Don't consciously let yourself fall on a slippery slope to average.

Think about lifting your grandkids and cavorting with them on a jungle gym like the agile and mobile kid you once were. How about unscrewing that tight bottle cap for your next of kin or playing better pickleball when your work-life balance allows? Ponder how you'll get that heavy suitcase out of the trunk or into the overhead bin without strain or pain. Or, perhaps as a family first responder, consider how you will physically support an elder parent, relative, friend or stranger in their ADLs.

Many quality-of-life enhancements happen when you are strong to save. *Period.* Let's review four die-harder-and-later enhancements for you.

1. **You improve your lasting capacity to handle your ADLs and stressful situations.**

Regular strenuous activity improves your down-aging potential. Moving stuff is a real, no-kidding regulator for your happy hormones like dopamine and also for your growth messengers like testosterone.

2. **You guard against premature sarcopenia *and* improve your skeletal health.**

You are a mammal, after all, with an endoskeleton that will serve you if you challenge it with weight-bearing motions.

3. **You metabolize calories effectively.**

Your physical activity impacts the number of calories you expend in your daily energy equations. The more active you are, the more calories you will burn during and after your strenuous exercise.

4. **You assuredly sleep better to allow scores of your bodily hormones to function as they should.**

Quality sleep is an absolute requirement to support the hundreds of hormonal processes that your body needs for proper physical banking. Serotonin is a vital one of those hundreds, as is testosterone for both sexes.

You should see clearly now. Your four types of D.E.E.P. strength, gained now or in the future, are cornerstone investments in your optimal health span and lifespan. Never forget that,

"Anyone, at any fitness level, can and should strength train. And it doesn't have to take hours at the gym to see results ... Grab a towel and get ready to feel strong."[20]

Since you grabbed your towel and you now feel strong, celebrate this chapter's selected strength move to feel strong and capable.

Grin and Bear it.

Be a student of this bodyweight quadruped or bear plank and progressive bear crawl. Be bear strong, like aesthetic Hollywood stars. Or emulate bear barbell workouts used by elite Paralympian rower, Todd Vogt, despite his early onset PD. As a great student, you can easily locate details of "stacked, complex" bear workouts that optimize your musculus' time under tension (TuT). Todd and I will applaud you.

Remember – safety first when you first tackle a bear.

And *bear* the strain in this regimen, like other great GenX athletes do.

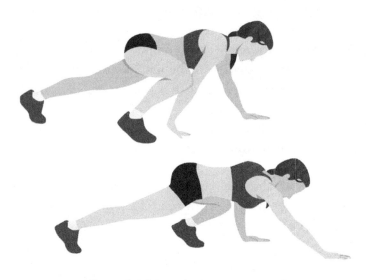

Figure 2.4 A Female GenX Bear Crawl

When you tap into the movement of the crawl's opposite-side arm and leg actions (see Figure 2.4), you improve your body's ability to move in many ADL situations—with superior balance and coordination. Plus, you can wear a weight vest or cleverly figure out other sources of additional weight to make these bear crawls more resistive.

FLEX ALERT #11:

It is imperative to preserve your ability to get up from the ground and confidently move around on the floor in your second half of life. Kid-like or bear-like floorwork notably reduces your risk of injuries from falls. You're engaging your upper body, core, and lower body at the same time.

Before you bear-crawl, consider an important flex check for your fall protection and longevity. It is called a sit-to-rise check, as shown in Figure 2.5. You rise from the floor without using your hands or supports. Whether this is initially easy or hard for you to execute, do get used to this check, please. It is a kid-like, complex move that requires strength and stability. Just be careful about slipping on throw rugs or waxed floors.

Check it out and perform it for many moons as a great GenX.

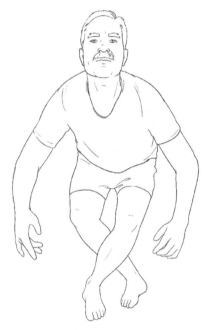

Figure 2.5 Your Sit-to-Rise Check for Longevity

Now, back to bear crawls.

URSA AND HOLLYWOOD ICONS ...

Be sure to brace your core muscle groups to stay low to the ground and keep your hips as level as possible. When your bear crawl or quadruped position is viewed from the side, your back should be flat like a table, and your knees should be *only* an inch or two off the ground.

Also, use your core muscles to combat excessive side-to-side rotation in your hips as you crawl. Stay balanced as you crawl in any of the four crawl directions—forward, back, left, and right. Some fitness professionals label crawls as longevity moves. *As a spoiler alert, you will read more about crawls as X factor movements in Chapter 8 of Strong to Save.*

WAIT WEIGHT

Your bear crawl *box routine* combines crawls in all four-corner directions. This challenges your strength, agility, and coordination in multiple directions. When you are loaded for bear, so to speak, you can also *overload* this awesome bodyweight exercise for strength and stability. You can carry a weighted plate or safely carry a grandkid on your level back during these Ursula moves. I suggest that you defer added-weight bear crawls until you can crawl in all four directions with good form for a minute.

TURN, TURN, TURN

Turn to chapter 3 for your source code that makes all else possible. With towel in hand and source code in mind, you do *not* need years of effort or buy expensive accessories to be strong to save.

Source Code

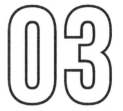

"Whatever your 100 percent looks like, *give it.*"

—Chyna Cho, CrossFit athlete

As a recognized CrossFit competitor, Chyna is a code breaker for a first principle of muscular achievement. Giving it all takes nearly all your sarcomeres in action with your mind-body alignment (MBA). Note: A 2011 sci-fi thriller *Source Code*, starring Jake Gyllenhaal, is *not* why this chapter is titled as it is.

Let's decode your programmed building blocks of skeletal muscle that enable you to give life a 100 percent effort, as Chyna implores you to. Leverage your source code of physical strength to deliver *whatever it takes* for your maximal performance today and for many tomorrows. Think of your sarcomeres as encoded filaments that will deliver strong after-effects. Remember the Rock's challenge to move what stands in your way—with situational all-out effort.

Your kinetic source code is embedded in about six hundred skeletal muscles and muscle groups. As you read earlier, Latin names for some muscles or groups are downright confusing. They frankly stress my mental capacity to memorize (and spell) muscles like:

- *Brachiradialus*
- *Infraspinatus*
- *Sternocleomastoid*
- *Pubococcygeus* muscle or PC

Note: This PC is pelvically correct. A well-developed *pubococcygeus* muscle can enhance sex and orgasm for both ladies and gentlemen. A strong PC muscle has also been linked to a reduction in urinary incontinence.[21]

- *Scalene posterior*
- *Levator veli pallatini* (one of my all-time funky favorites.)

I cautioned you about arcane Greek and Latin names for muscles and muscle groups, didn't I?

It is more important to exercise your source code than to spell a sourced muscle correctly. So, celebrate our capacity to use nicknames—like *hammies and lats, quads and calves, or delts* and *traps*—plus acronyms like TVA and TFL or IO instead of full muscle names. Celebrate core motions like hip abduction or leg adduction without knowing the many muscle groups that serve as those motions' agonists and antagonists.

Drumroll: Your well-developed muscles help you work wonders. Let's uncover their source.

Your many marvelous motions are *not* triggered by *digital* source code. Muscle movement is triggered *chemically* and *electrically* rather than as binary or hexadecimal computer coding in our information age. Your wondrous central nervous system (CNS), that includes the brain and spinal column, chemically triggers your neuromuscular systems with electrical impulses.[22] Think of your peak neuromuscular interactions as firing on all cylinders.

CODE?

I don't insist, and neither do I encourage you to chase down the known facts of neurotransmitters like acetylcholine, the intra-cellular pumping roles of calcium and sodium, or the secretive machinations of our CNS.

Remember that I cautioned against chasing the secrets of how sarcomeres work—that is, unless you like to emulate Alice in her Wonderland's futile chases.

Peripheral nervous system (PNS) cells communicate throughout our bodies after receiving CNS signals. Twelve cranial nerves, including the uber-important *vagus* as your tenth cranial nerve, make your gut and "guns" fire in concert. Doesn't that make you think of AC/DC energies?

Now is a perfect time to reinforce the importance of nervous system tune-ups so that your mind and muscle spindles function as best they can. Yes, you can strengthen your neuromuscular system using all-natural techniques mentioned by Cynthia Cross:

✓ Breathe mindfully and deeply.
✓ Bond with Mother Earth by going barefoot.
✓ Absorb and process natural vitamin D (from the sun).
✓ Try Yoga—formally or informally.
✓ Exercise regularly (duh).
✓ Absorb magnesium via Epsom salt soaks, natural foods, or well-chosen and trusted supplements.
✓ Absorb those wonderful water-soluble vitamin Bs (from natural food sources when possible).
✓ Ingest "good" fatty acids—particularly omega-3s, *not* omega-6 fatty acids.
✓ Drink green tea or take trusted green tea supplements to boost your happy chemical messaging (serotonin and dopamine).
✓ Change up your workouts (remember what I S.A.I.D.).
✓ Visualize your performance and get into a "flow zone."[23]

Right, when you actively think about your effort and (silently) talk to your muscles, you improve your mind-muscle connection and performance. I jest not, so please use regular private communiques to stimulate your muscles or "little mice."

If you train with me, you'll often hear me encourage you to squeeze and activate your gluteal muscles and flatten your belly button to your backbone or spine. Are you using your breathing rhythm to your advantage? Are you in a performance zone with an aligned mind and body? When you get into a flow zone with these prompts, your mind and body are better aligned for D.E.E.P. muscular performance. Your spatial awareness, or proprioception, is enhanced too.

HOW ABOUT TUNES?

I won't delve in music as a feel-good enabler for performance. Suffice it to state that researchers have proof that music can aid in workouts. If you do listen to tunes in a gym or public place, please be considerate of others.

Sthenic source codes are depicted here for a GenX in *safe*, dynamic motion (see Figure 3.1.)

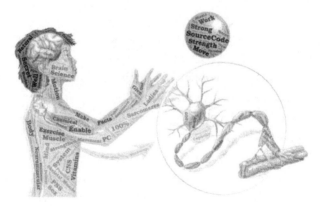

Figure 3.1 Source Codes at Work via Mind Body connections

SAFETY FIRST

Be prudent and be safe for all of your progressive strength and resistance activities. As many health organizations advise, "Check with your doctor to make sure it's safe for you to proceed." Amen.

√ Gain your MD's approval before you engage in strenuous strength routines. It is fine to start bodyweight exercises to personally gauge your strength before you see the doctor. She or he may evaluate how you hip-hinge to rise from a chair in your consultative visit, so practice, practice, practice. Practice good-morning (bobbing bird) stretches, air squats, and straight-leg deadlifts without weights as your personal readiness assessments.

It is better to be safe than sorry as another platitude that you've heard. Learn to appreciate the difference in your neuromuscular feedback signals. There is a key difference between muscle soreness (DOMS) and joint discomfort or pain. Exercise-induced muscle soreness is expected, yet joint or connective tissue pains are a different matter. It is always best to record aches and pains, right? Please journal your body's feedback in context of your workouts, and please do not push through pain. A great GenX is a great recording star.

YOUR PHYSICAL APTITUDE READINESS-QUESTIONNAIRE

You may have seen or completed a physical aptitude readiness questionnaire (PAR-Q)[24] before you worked with a fitness trainer like me. This *health-and-wellness* checklist is mandatory for older (sixty-plus) athletes. If you have hypertension, the types of strength activities that you do should be tuned with high blood pressure in mind. Of the D.E.E.P. types of strength, noted earlier, those with hypertension should be wary of **p**eak power and **e**xplosive (plyometric) work. Conversely, **e**ndured strength can be safely pursued by walking with wrist weights. The *notorious* Supreme Court Judge Ruth Bader Ginsburg still worked her **d**ynamic strength with light weights after her multiple cancer bouts in elder years.

I hope that I piqued your interest about intersecting lifestyle factors and strengths to save at any age. Repeat after me as your strength coach: *power begins with knowledge.* Know the odds to beat the odds to *stay stronger for longer.*

Please complete these physical readiness checks and situationally revisit them to monitor your trends:

- ✓ Easily evaluate your physical bank portfolio with an anonymous online estimator called the Living to 100 calculator. Dr. Thomas Perls devised this credible application to help you identify personal choices to live longer and better.
- ✓ Learn about your atherosclerotic cardiovascular disease (ASCVD) risks for the next decade of your life. I repeat: CVD is the leading cause of mortality for American adults. (I could also restate that cancers are the third leading cause of American adult mortality. There are credible links between cancer and poor lifestyle diets and exercise. Yet let's address Public Enemy #1 first.)

- Find the reputable American Heart Association's (AHA) online estimator for lifespan risks. Candidly respond with your vital inputs. Then start to beat actuarial odds with knowledge and awareness.

- Search online for the Mayo Clinic's credible calculator for long-term risks for CVD. Data entry parameters for it are longer and a shade different than the AHA's just mentioned tool (including your weekly physical exertion.) Yet, these extra keystrokes efforts are not burdensome. Note: This Mayo Clinic estimation is very consistent with the AHA estimator in my case.

    As Mark Twain challenged authors like me, "Write what you know." I know and share my CV risk (meaning a potential heart attack or stroke), and I know how to reduce my risks. According to these AHA and Mayo Clinic estimators, plus my MD consultations, I now carry a 12 to 13 percent physical and medical risk of having a CV event in my next decade. Can I do better? Yup. Am I working on these credible action items (below) to reduce my risk? Yes, I am with simple lifestyle choices that complement my strength regimens:

- Commit to an anti-inflammatory, healthy (lifestyle) diet:
    o Eat rainbow colors regularly—fruits, vegetables, and whole grains.
    o Eat red meat sparingly. Pick alternatives, low-fat dairy products, and organic poultry, certain fish, and legumes.
    o Eat moderate amounts of healthy fats, such as unsalted nuts and omega-3 oils.
- Forego smoking cigarettes/cigars or using tobacco products—always.
- Reduce the total number of calories in your daily diet. Think of just one daily beer, a glass of wine, or a spirit shot as a monthly *pound* of calories to account for in your energy equations. Whether you imbibe or not is up to you. Just remember that even "light beer" or "skinny" wine drinks can have fatty consequences on your middle-age journey.

Let me serve as a canary in a coal mine to warn of life-cheating factors that you can control! Floss your teeth, moderate your daily caffeine consumption, even if it is green tea and organic coffee, and always wear your seat belt.

Shifting from canary to champion, I move heavy stuff twice each week in dedicated strength regimes. And I build my stamina with at least 450 minutes of endured strength activities in each and every week. Yes, this equates to many, many MET minutes weekly. Next, I add one more longevity estimator.

UBER-FIT NORWEGIANS

Please take the authoritative fitness age calculation steps developed by a Norwegian University's Cardiac Exercise Research Group (CERG) at this website: https://www.worldfitnesslevel.org/#/.

Embrace the worth of these two strong, reputable quotes from Viking land:

1. "The four most important factors for fitness ... namely age, waist circumference, leisure-time physical activity and resting heart rate—are those included in the algorithm that constitutes our Fitness Calculator ..."

2. "The estimated fitness number is of great importance for how long you can expect to live. That's why we now recommend every physician to use the calculator to identify patients with a high risk of lifestyle diseases and early death."[25]

    Notes: a. It is not just for physicians. Every great GenX should use this critical calculator too. b. I trust that you highlighted *waist circumference* among the four parameters for this longevity calculator.

SAY WHAT?

I underscore this Norwegian cardio challenge with some facts. The Norway University of Science and Technology (NTNU in our English translation) has researched fitness ages for more than six million adults. Shouldn't you add to this information base too?

- The average man has a fitness number of 50.4 by the valid "macro" CERG calculations.
    - o I am blessed, and I do the work to have the estimated fitness of a twenty-nine- to thirty-one-year-old male with

my NTNU Fitness Number of 52. Now, find yours as a sharp student of your endeavors. Then move it, move it.

- The average woman in the CERG "big data" analyses has a fitness number of 40.6.
- The average man sits 7.2 hours a day. Do you?
- The average woman sits 6.8 hours a day. Do you?

Are you ready for my punchline about your source code? Here 'tis:

Regular physical activity *eliminates* the increased risk associated with a sedentary lifestyle.

Even among sedentary adults, those who exercise had significantly higher cardiovascular capacity (aka VO_2 max) than individuals who did not. Duh—motion is medicine. I underscore that:

> your resistance training contributes to a
> lower fitness age calculation.

KNOW YOUR NUMBERS

Know your body's current kinetic capacities to lift, push, pull, twist, and carry objects. Know how, when, and why to move heavy stuff and sweat. Know how to time and fuel your workouts. Grasp what restore, replenish, and rebuild practices work best for you at this time. Knowledge is power. Knowledge is your safe and sound requisite for optimal physical banking.

- ✓ Record your key body measurements and analyze your trends.
- ✓ Know your body type and what it takes to win in the strength game of life.

It is imperative to start, extend, and expand on what you can and will do! Don't chase an impossible dream of becoming "the Rock," yet attain a possible dream of being *strong as the new skinny*.

Don't pass through a door of discomfort to get an extra repetition or move extra tonnage. Discomfort and pain are feedback to which you must listen. Know your current power and strength for moves like the deadweight lift. Be in the Know to give 100%.

RE-MEM-MEM, RE-MEM-ME-MEM-BER

✓ Remember how to leverage these science-backed and sweat-based principles for your fitness age and down-aging.
✓ Remember that each GenX athlete is different, and so is her or his source code's natural regeneration. "If you have a body, you are an athlete" (Bill Bowerman, coach, and cofounder of Nike®).

What about that amazing body of yours? There is a longstanding and somewhat philosophical debate for influences of genetic and environmental factors on longevity. In two influential words, *nature* and *nurture*.

"Nature refers to all of the genes and hereditary factors that influence who we are—from our physical appearance to our personality characteristics."

"Nurture refers to all the environmental variables that impact who we are, including our early childhood experiences, how we were raised, our social relationships, and our surrounding culture."[26]

WHAT DO YOU CONTROL?

Some aspects of obesity and poor fitness are assuredly genetic and prewired for you at birth. That's nature (and about *fifty* human hormones) at work or misworking. Yet it is a *minority* factor for your physical banking. Other aspects of obesity and poot fitness are sadly enabled by fast foods, sedentary lifestyles, and poorly tuned biochemical factors. That is nurture, but nurture that is *not* working well. And sadly, this is your majority factor for staying decent or just staying good as a GenX.

The extension to be a great GenX is to eat clean, avoid sedentary practices at work and leisure, and to tune up your source code to gain that added decade of health span.

It is a bit late to recruit new parents by nature. You should rather focus on nurturing your health span and lifespan habits for success. Yes, you can and should acknowledge some blessings or curses that were passed down to you. Here is a newsflash that is so obvious that I did not label it as a Flex Alert:

It is better to nurture yourself with positive "down-aging" than to concede to bell-curve aging from nature.

Do not blame your forebears. *Do* nurture your physical bank and strong cornerstone. You do not need to concede to the *im*moral majority of nature.

In her book *The Body Myth*, Dr. Margo Maine writes that people often mistake health for weight and body shapes. Our weight and body shape can be health concerns, but they are not absolute indicators of health.[27]

Remember your athlete within, then knowledgeably and continually play the hand you are dealt by both nature and nature. If you are heavy, train for functional strength. If you are not great and have a lean ectomorph body type, then train for functional strength anyway. If you are intent on dying harder and later, lift for functional strength. I know you see my emphases on functional strength, right? Functional strengths support activities of everyday life.

Down-aging can be yours with great functional strength, although you won't reach the reported age of a certain biblical patriarch.

WHO WAS METHUSELAH?

An Old Testament patriarch named Methuselah *supposedly* lived long—as in very long—as in *centuries* long. Fascination with healthy aging and long lifespans is very much in our current news. Fountains of youth are going viral in social media channels these days. Anti-aging quests promote "big pharma" sales of more and costlier "geroprotection" drugs than ever before. Please note that Methuselah *didn't* have a Medicare card for polypharmacy or geroprotection drugs. He didn't know or care about epigenetics.

Neither did the world's oldest living person of 122 verified years – a French lady named Jeanne Calment – so why should you? 'Tis sad yet true that Americans are prescribed and take "therapeutic" drugs at what I call alarming rates and quantities. An average GenX takes 2 or more prescription pills daily. If those pills are lifesaving for sick care, I'm okay. If those pills are not prescribed for life-saving reasons, I am not okay with *over* prescriptions for "health care." In that same bible that cites Methuselah, there is a saying to honor your body like a temple. I like that honor code.

Healthy aging works better for others in the animal kingdom than it does for us. I cite a recent (2022) book titled *Methuselah's Zoo* by Steven Austad. You may recognize Dr. Austad as half of the Billion Dollar wager for longevity that was conceived with his colleague Dr. Olshansky in 2001. That longevity wager is quite fascinating, as is an active read of *Methuselah's Zoo*. Austad stresses that we have much to learn from nature about longevity and aging—like sharks, *immortal* amoebas (no kidding), and bristlecone pine trees. I'll try to do justice to Dr. Austad's double bottom line:

Those species or individuals that can:

a. avoid environmental dangers or hazards and
b. limit aging cancers (as cell division run amok) to die harder and later. Period.

You can tackle longevity of animal kingdom outliers as another interesting homework assignment. Let's shift back to Homo sapiens and our regeneration for lifespan and health span. Austad confirms that we are the longest living mammals walking on earth. Yet he questions why some birds and sea creatures dodge cancer, still mate late in life, and thrive in harsh conditions. Let us consider normal cell division or regeneration, also known as autophagy.

REGENERATION?

Scientists report that 1–2 percent of our muscles' myonuclei are regenerated each week. Yup. Your skeletal muscles are replaced by bodily autophagy every few months en toto. *Autophagy* literally means a self-eating, recycling system. Incidentally, I commend to you *The Power of Autophagy* by Douglas Tieman.

Two other relevant recycling facts are: Your entire blood capacity is renewed every calendar quarter as a natural "pro survival" process. And even your amazing cardiovascular pump, that smooth operator or left ventricle of your heart, does a complete changeout every forty-eight to sixty months. Talk about makeovers…

Here is your sixty-four-thousand-dollar question that might need to be adjusted for today's inflation (in 2023):

What activities stimulate cellular renewal that doesn't run amok?

One of four very powerful answer starts and ends with the letter *E* - *Exercise*. Three other "green recycling" efforts for potential longevity are 1.) fasting, 2.)caloric restriction, and 3.) carbohydrate restriction (aka ketogenics.)

I add two other books to chew and digest thoroughly if you are interested in thought leadership on longevity matters.

1. A GenX doctor and podcast host, Peter Attia, released (2023) *Outlive: The Science and Art of Longevity.*

2. A very fine GenX author, Steven Johnson, released (in 2021) *Extra Life: A Short History of Living Longer.*

FLEX ALERT #12:

Exercise is a natural, effective way to promote cellular renewal and to offset senescence (as seen in Figure 3.2).[28]

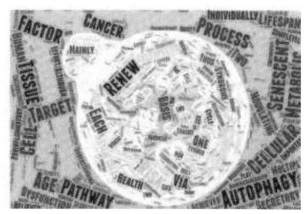

Figure 3.2 Cellular Renewal

Senescence, huh? Get this, *senescence* comes from the Latin root *senex*, which also relates to senile and senate. You can look that up in your *Funk and Wagnalls*, or *Merriam-Webster Dictionary.*

Senescence is our "normal" aging process. "Normal" aging cells lose their vitality, yet some or many don't get replaced by autophagy. Senescent cells can be thought of as zombie cells that hang around and clog up your system, in a way like dirty old sludge clogs up your car's oil lubricants. I don't like zombie anything. Do you?

What's a GenX to do about senescence? Take note: You can voluntarily control your sludge buildup by doing some or all of the *four* recycling activities that I just cited to limit your own nights of the living dead. How about a wee bit of cellular biology with DNA replication to cap things off?

CAP OFF CODING

'Tis fascinating that your exercise lengthens *telomere* caps of your cells' DNA strands or laces. This equates to longer cell life before senescence. You can trust Nobel prize winners on this phenomenon. Longer telomeres come *only* from extended space travel or exercise. Exercise can and should be hard, yet it is much easier and cheaper than space travel with Elon Musk. Improved cellular health, meet longer telomeres lengthened by exercise.[29]

Amanda Macmillan, a *TIME* reporter, stated: "Telomeres ... are markers of aging and overall health. A tiny bit of telomere is lost every time a cell replicates, so they get shorter with age. People who exercised the most had significantly longer telomeres than those who were sedentary. People who did vigorous exercise had telomeres that signaled about seven fewer years of biological aging, compared to people who did moderate levels of activity."[30] Exercise lengthens telomeres to downage your cells!

Dwell on that fact. Seven *or more* years can be your savings to thrive and strive after halftime. Twenty-five hundred extra sunrises and days of wonder to cherish in those seven downaged years. Yes, you may recall that I suggest, and I believe in about ten years of down-aging in other *Strong to Save* pages. I like the prospect of an extra 2500 to 3652 healthy sunrises, don't you? Now read how a clean dietary lifestyle with big and little nutrients fits into your kinetic counts, muscular source codes, proper lifts, and longer health span.

MACROS AND MICROS

I'm not double-talking here, so please bear with me to address big and little, or macro- and micro nutrients. Great exercise is invaluable for your physical retirement account. Yet, a great GenX *cannot* thrive by exercise alone. There is a dietary imperative to eat cleanly, almost always, to sustain your strong-to-save efforts. Why?

Your exercise causes oxidation as a byproduct, a "free radical," or a reactive oxygen species (ROS) in biochemical parlance. That free radical will easily combine with other molecules to damage and age one's cellular DNA—*if* you allow that "rust" to accumulate. *Isn't it ironic that oxygen is life for us, yet it can also lead to rusty disease and death?* Note: **Cancer** was what Dr. Austad called "cell division run amok" with aging. That is the same principle as rusty disease and premature death from oxidative free radicals. Of course, I implore you to exercise, though you create short-lived rust and inflammation when you do.

To counter bodily rust and oxidative effects, you must put biochemistry to work for you as natural geroprotection. You will neutralize oxidants as radical, reactive rust with the *anti*oxidants you absorb. And I hope that you naturally get as many of these life-extending antioxidants from Vitamin P, for plants, and adaptogens for herbs, rather than from un-regulated supplements. Please highlight my down-aging platitude to

"eat *all* colors of the rainbow daily."

Rainbows of Vitamin P are like your Rustoleum™ warranty that can lead you to a pot of seven to ten more golden years. Yes, there are plenty of antioxidants that you can purchase as dietary supplements—from exotic krill to astaxanthin to some fish oils.

- Strive to absorb as much of your antioxidant needs from natural complete foods as you can.

Better absorption of vital nutrients is one reason to focus on clean eating of natural and hopefully organic food. Let's move on to your cellular building blocks, your very own living LEGOS™ blocks or elements.

IT'S ELEMENTARY, WATSON

Believe it or not, my dear Watson, just six elements make up about 94 percent of your body mass. That is correct, *oxygen, carbon, hydrogen, nitrogen, calcium*, and *sodium* are your super six elements.

The remaining 6 percent of your elemental mass is important for your health span and lifespan as well. Think of these vital *micro* minerals: sulfur, selenium, chromium, magnesium, potassium, and phosphorus. You should gain at least a bit of practical information about your mineral rights to appreciate *the full Monty*—or 100 percent—of your biochemical makeup to skirt danger.

DANGER ZONE

Warning signs for *peligro* or danger are to be avoided, of course. I cite selected dietary no-no's that can adversely impact your health span. Avoid them or limit their daily intakes:

- Zombie or hidden fats in mayonnaise, French fries, fast-food hamburgers, deep-fried chips, milk chocolate, pastries, and crusted pies.
- Excessively charred foods from your grill.
- Cured cold cuts and meat (the sodium nitrites and nitrates used for processing and preserving may be unhealthy. Conversely, nitrates and nitrites in vegetables like celery and cucumbers are *not*.)
- Simple sugars and "super-sized" high fructose corn syrup drinks. Fitness oriented women should limit total carbohydrates to about 50 grams per day (note that healthy fiber is also classified as a carbohydrate, so *don't* shortchange healthy fiber.) Fit men can consume up to 100 grams a day of carbohydrates to fuel their muscles rather than fill their white

fat cells. Note that these strong-to-save recommendations diverge from our government's suggested daily intakes.*

- Sodium—just a teaspoon (~2.3 grams)—is adequate for you each day. Most adults get 1½ to 2 teaspoons each day because of processed convenient foods. Excess oy!
- Inflammatory, high omega-6 products (grain-fed meat products, processed vegetable oils like sunflower, corn, soybean, and cottonseed oil.)
- Monosodium glutamate (MSG) as a flavor enhancer.
- Possible testosterone-limiting factor (TLF) foods. Juries are still out on the long-term health effects of foods like soy, licorice root, and mint. I limit my intake of these TLFs, and I definitely shy away from vegetable oils and processed foods at least six days each week. - Please apply a prudent 80/20 rule for clean eating as I do. Yes, it is OK, and may actually be beneficial—for you to stray from clean eating one a day a week. Okay, one day doesn't exactly equal 20 percent, yet you get my drift for a slack day each week.
- Artificial additives. Try to find natural sweeteners and flavor enhancers as healthy alternatives to almost anything artificial.
- Bisphenol A (BPA) in packaging and plastics. Though our FDA states that BPA is safe in "small doses," it is best to go with BPA-free products. *Who wants industrial chemicals in your food or drink?*

Footnote*: Let me repeat my aggressive daily macro-nutrient benchmarks for GenX women and men who choose to be lean, great, and strong.

- Carbohydrates (including fiber):
  - Women should strive to limit their daily carbohydrate intake to a total of 50 grams.

- o   Being larger and carrying more vital tissues like muscles, men should strive to limit their daily carbohydrate intake to 100 grams.
- Fats: Both women and men should strive to eat ½ gram of *healthy* fats per pound of bodyweight daily
- Proteins: Both women and men should strive to eat one (1) gram of complete protein per pound of bodyweight daily. This goal is admittedly tough as this amounts to a lot of chicken breasts, or eggs, or Greek yogurt.

First, I don't want you to go overboard to meet or beat these tough benchmark levels for macronutrients. Yet, keep in mind that you will suffer sarcopenia if you only eat what our Government suggests is your daily guideline for being decent or average. I implore you to do your best.

Second, I don't want you to go overboard with *total* avoidance of these danger zone products. Satchel Paige's advisory about *moderation* can serve you well. He meant that it was OK to enjoy a very occasional hot dog at the ballpark—as in, not too many, and not too often. Use that clean 80/20 guideline: Holiday treats of prudent portions can be forgiven if you get back on the natural and healthy lifestyle train quickly. Be as natural as you can to cultivate a healthy gut and limit bodily inflammation as best you can.

I recall the advice of one respected researcher who said to get your clean diet right most of the time, but *not* to strive for always right.

Repeat after me if you *are* interested in living long and well:

1. I will absorb naturally sourced vitamins, which are *essential* for my normal cell function, growth, and development.
2. I will ingest and absorb key minerals and compounds to keep my bones, muscles, heart, and brain working properly.
3. I will naturally *manufacture* needed enzymes and hormones to keep me strong, stable, and supple for about fifty more quality years.

MIGHTY MICROS

You know micronutrients are smaller than macros, yes? You hopefully know how critical "micros" are for your quest to live long and well. Think minerals and think vitamins or plant compounds from fertile soil. Avoid these micronutrients at your peril. Avoidance or sub-nourishment as I call it leads to oxidative rust that leads to inflammation and probably leads to cancer for a normal GenX. Face nourishment as a truth and consequence.

I commend a Center for Disease Control reference for dietary vitals that are small yet *mighty*:

"vital to development, disease prevention, and well-being. Micronutrients are *not* produced in the body and must be derived from your diet. Deficiencies in micronutrients, such as iron, iodine, vitamin A, folate, and zinc can have devastating consequences."[31]

Don't be *devastated* by sub-nourishment, but don't go overboard with them either.

Do you remember Mae West? I can't find fault with some of her alluring thoughts, yet I do in this case of micronutrients. Too much of a good thing may *not* be wonderful. Intentional or unintentional "overdosing" of some micronutrients *doesn't* improve the credit rating of your physical bank. Iron is one mineral to moderate, and fat-soluble vitamins (A,D E, and K) can build up if taken excessively. So don't "*OD*" on D or other micronutrients. Let's change gears.

It is important to review certain medical challenges and physical conditions. In your Strong to Save Introduction, I cited my intent for an inclusive fit map. I want nearly all GenX to strive toward impeccable performance. I laud the efforts of Todd Vogt and others who keep walking through hell. Keep motion, even if it is modified motion, as your very good medicine. Never quit, not now or ever.

STAT

Bear with me now. Yes, this paragraph's title, "Stat," is from the Latin word *statim*, which means *now*. My quick synopses of deadly or life altering conditions herein are neither authoritative nor in-depth. Yet, I cite them because exercise can *put the brakes on* these challenged athlete conditions in many cases. Motion and resistance training are *very* good medicine.

First, consider some conditions that can chip away at one's sense-and-respond neuromuscular system. Although these conditions affect only a minority of GenX, one of that minority might be an acquaintance, a family member, or it could be you.

Neuromuscular disorders (NMD) impair voluntary muscle functions that may cause a loss of motile function or movement. If nerves of your CNS get affected, become senescent, or die, then your nervous system fails to communicate effectively with the intended bodily muscles. Without activation, those skeletal muscles may weaken, shrink, and waste away. One's motion as good medicine is threatened.

One sad NMD is Parkinson's disease or PD. You may recognize PD from its sad effects on boxer Muhammad Ali, actor Michael J. Fox, and Pope John Paul II. Uncurable sad effects include advancing tremors, limb rigidity, wobbly gait, and balance problems. You now know from these pages how strength has helped an elite "para" athlete and rower, Todd Vogt, deal with his early onset of PD. TINA for him, or for others.

FLEX ALERT #13:

Increasing physical activities early in life will lower the risk of developing PD later in life.[32]

Another neuromuscular and autoimmune disease / disorder is multiple sclerosis (MS). This disease or disorder can affect one's brain and spinal cord, vision, arm or leg movement, sensation, or balance. As an autoimmune disease, MS somehow causes one's body to attack itself and to increase its chronic inflammations. *Some types of arthritis are also autoimmune disorders.* Causes of MS are unfortunately unclear, as was the case for PD. Exercise programs are recommended under the guidance of a physiotherapist to counter some effects of MS.[33]

Another neuromuscular disorder that affects *too many* adults is muscular dystrophy (MD). This is an inherited disease that damages and weakens skeletal muscles over time. It is caused by the deficiency of a protein called dystrophin. Sadly, like other NMDs, there is no current cure for MD. Please, please, please play the hand you're dealt to be the best that you can be, whatever disorder or NMD confronts you.

It is time to examine another strong move to counter inflammation and for some, to counter NMD.

EUREKA!

You've now come across this chapter's strength move, the hip flex, that is also known as a glute bridge as illustrated in Figure 3.3:

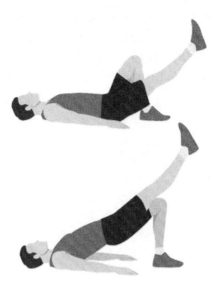

Figure 3.3 A Male GenX Unilateral
Glute Bridge (Bodyweight).

This unilateral (one-sided) hip flex or glute bridge is more advanced than a bilateral (symmetrical) move of the same name. You get the picture?

1. Lie flat on the floor or a yoga mat, breathing mindfully and tucking your belly button to your backbone.
2. Bring your heels toward your hips as close as is comfortable for you.
3. Squeeze your glutes and compress your "hip flexor" psoas muscles to lift your hips off the ground.
4. Lower your hips to the ground slowly for one repetition.
   o You can add a weighted bar across your hips or place a weighted plate on your front hip crest for an advanced glute bridge. *Remember that your glutes are uber-powerful when activated.* Thus, as a strong GenX, you should be able to perform the glute bridge with a heavy weighted bar or plate or with a special workout buddy straddling you.

Yes, your upper legs and lower back also benefit from this exercise that promotes strong "core work" for other weight lifts and activities. Are you ready to move on to twigs, rodents, and muscle talk? I'm playfully serious. Please turn your page to learn about strong "little mice."

Strong "Little Mice"

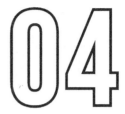

"A single twig breaks, but the bundle of twigs is strong."

—Tecumseh, Shawnee chief, and warrior

Congratulations. You are pressing to become *Strong to Save* and are working to die harder. Now, you can talk about the king or queen of lifts—the deadlift. You know kinetic numbers or counts to beat actuarial odds by moving stuff as very good medicine. As a spoiler alert, you will soon be ready to Sexercise as more good medicine. And you can always refer to your dog-eared and highlighted pages to cite Flex Alerts from your fitmat—PRN.

This chapter's twiggy epigraph, attributed to a legendary Native American warrior, should resonate. If his words *do not* resonate, please pass this book to someone who grips the importance of strong bundles. Let's flex our verbal knowledge of the keyword, strength, one more time.

From old Germanic roots, *strength* means bodily power, force, vigor, firmness, or fortitude. Strong, the first word in your book title, also has similar old English origins.

Please act on your word knowledge to build strength as a firm cornerstone in your physical banking efforts. Examine the firm grip of Figure 4.1 as a think piece for bundles of strength and power generation:

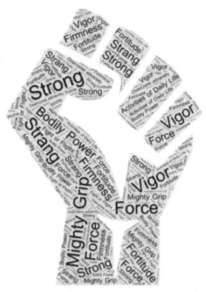

Figure 4.1 Your Strong "Little Mice" Chapter Themes

Begin lifting, pushing, pulling, carrying, and twisting for a longer healthy life with your gathered knowledge of "little mice."

You read that correctly, *little mice*. You can and should flex your "musculus" or *little mice* as did Romans in days of yore. We credit the French with using the word "muscle" for the first time about eight hundred years ago. Get ready to show off those bundles, flex those little mice, and move your body today and for many tomorrows.

Let's consider your prime movers.

Your amazing body brandishes three muscle tissue types:

1. **Smooth**
2. **Cardiac**
3. **Striated** or **skeletal** fibers.

✓ Your smooth gut muscles are certainly important. Their smooth operations support digestive processes to refuel your vital organs like muscles. They also stand as a garden wall around your microbiome to limit "leaky gut" inflammations into your body. A Red Flag! If your gut is misbehaving, your resistance training is likely suffering.

✓ Your heart's left ventricle is a critically important *cardiac* muscle. It contracts with each of your heartbeats to pulse oxygen and glucose through thousands of miles of your vascular pipelines to nourish your organs and muscles. This cardiac muscle is a key enabler for longevity in the Norwegian CERG model. By the way, when I wrote thousands of miles, I was conservative as you have about *60,000 miles* of piping in your amazing body.

✓ Unless otherwise specified, the term "muscle" in *Strong to Save* represents a human's *striated skeletal* muscle or *sarcomere*. Now, remember what Tecumseh wrote about bundles.

KINETIC CONNECTION

"Skeletal muscle fibers are bound together by connective tissue and communicate with nerves and blood vessels."[34]

Why do I stress this point? As a systems engineer by first profession, I share systematic relationships and interactions that make motion your medicine. You are functionally strong when your tendons, ligaments, fascia, and joints collaborate with muscle fibers to bear life's strains for your impeccable second-half performance. As you may know or will learn from these pages, your intrabody collaborations for locomotion have biochemical and biomechanical features and functions to appreciate and leverage.

Your evolved skeletal muscles, along with other muscle groups give your human form its structural shape for "standup" results: "(human) life evolved in the presence of gravity, and it has long been recognized, … that posture is maintained by tonic muscle contractions acting against gravity and stabilizing the positions of body segments …"[35]

Parenthetically, earthly gravity is also the force that stimulates skeletal strength. Now, you may agree that my introductory explanation for the features and functions of skeletal muscle is complex and can be confounding. You are *not* alone. "Recent biochemical and biomechanical findings have forced a serious reevaluation of structural and functional muscle complexity." [36]

Let's avoid a sarcomere swamp, at least until science simplifies how our complex muscles truly work. Now, just focus on flexing and extending your skeletal muscle fibers to move bodily joints. And it is a great GenX tactic to add playfulness to your ADLs.

FLEX ALERT #14:

Laughter is a good medicinal complement for strength building. Your sense of humor just may help you keep on keepin' on when the going gets tough in a strength session or activity.

Consider these three chuckles as you flex and extend sarcomeres:

1. My average leg day is doing diddly *squat.*[37]
2. Why did the blonde get a perm?

   Because her personal trainer said, "*Curls* might help you."[38]

3. As author Judith Vorst suggested, "Strength is the ability to break a chocolate into four pieces and eat only one."

Smile, then repeat after me to make the grade.

D.E.E.P. THINKING AND DOING

It is your prime time to regrip those four types of human strength:

Impressive human strength that is enabled by six hundred muscle groups. Be an *A* student in physical education for these D.E.E.P. and powerful classes:

1. Dynamic
2. Elastic
3. Endured
4. Peak.

I assure you that we will hit plenty of repetitions for each type of strength. I also guarantee that volume, intensity, and tempo parameters of your moves to get and stay strong will be emphasized. Kinetics *do* count.

MUSCLE MOVES

Two types of muscle contractions —*isotonic* and *isometric*— help you build up and sustain your muscles size and function. Isometric contractions and flexions *do not* move joints. Isotonic contractions do move a joint or joints, as you can imagine for common weight lifts or resistance moves.

I appreciate isometric exercise—like a wall sit or a quadruped plank. So should you. Strong sumo wrestlers make some of their livelihood by standing their ground. For completeness, the period between a muscle's contraction and extension is called the isometric period of a repetition or move as shown earlier in Figure 1.1. This stationary period can be at the bottom, or at the top of a resistance move, perhaps a biceps curl or a chin-up. Do remember that isometrics can be done anywhere and without heavy metal. Now that you've noted isometric practices, move to the more recognized strength movements.

ISOTONIC MOVEMENT

An isotonic movement involves the contraction of one (or more) muscle(s) to move a skeletal joint through a partial or full range of motion or ROM. Consider an isotonic biceps curl like the one shown in Figure 4.2:

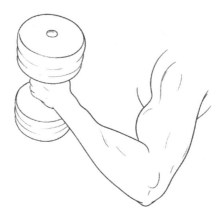

Figure 4.2 Isotonic Contraction in a Biceps Curl

When you perform that biceps curl, you "isotonically" contract forearm, upper arm, shoulder, and back muscle fibers to create a force against the gripped weight. As your activated muscle fibers shorten, your elbow joint ranges in motion to lift the forearm and your gripped dumbbell weight. That is one repetition. We'll skip over the Latin names of the many muscles involved in this isolation weight lift. That is, unless you need to know *brachioradialis* for a spelling bee.

Here is another example of a most important movement, the Air Squat, with compliments to *Outside* magazine.[39]

- ✓ Stand tall with your feet shoulder-width apart and your toes pointed forward. (Yes, there are variations of the basic squat for your feet and arms positions.)
- ✓ Hold your chest and head high (a neutral neck is important), pull your shoulders back and down, and engage your core muscles. (Think of pulling your belly button in toward your spine.)
- ✓ Bend your knees, and hinge slightly forward at the hips as if you're sitting down in a chair.
- ✓ Hold your arms out in front of you for counterbalance if needed. Continue lowering, keeping your angled back straight

and your torso upright until your thighs are nearly parallel to the ground or as far as you can with good form.

✓ Engage your glutes and push through your heels to stand for one repetition.

I again skip over the many muscles and muscle groups involved in this complex isotonic muscle move—the air squat. Full knowledge of those little mice and bundled twigs is important to a PhD of kinesiology. Yet perfect knowledge won't hinder you or help you to be stronger. There are many strong folks who do not know Latin, I assure you.

FLEX ALERT #15:

Learn to love your squats and perform them daily.

Why? Your strong legs, glutes and back muscles, hip hinge/ mobility, ankle flexion, and balance are true enablers for your many activities of daily life (ADL.) Testosterone (T) levels gets boost as well. I *stress* the importance of strength and stability as your practical accident insurance to avoid falls in your years ahead.

Activities of daily life and exercises—like walking, running, hiking, swimming, skiing, and dancing—are isotonic exercises. Movements such as the just-mentioned squat plus a biceps curl, push-up, pull-up, bench press, and your royal deadlift (from chapter 1), are also isotonic movements. Why? You force your skeletal joint(s) through ranges of motion (RoM). Isotonic exercise should *not* be a chore or a bore. Vary your exercise motion as a way to play while you get essential exercise[40] throughout your second half of life. Now, think about other benefits.

Isotonic movements also strengthen your cardiovascular system, boost your oxygen (O2) consumption, heart stroke volume, and muscular endurance for both type I (slow twitch) and type 2 (fast twitch) fibers.

Ladies, please highlight the known fact that weight-bearing exercise can help you stave off "osteo" problems. Ladies and gentlemen, your strong movements boost your metabolism and improve cholesterol and blood sugar levels. Most importantly, isotonics help you resist injury from strains, sprains, fractures, and falls. One more stationary rep...

ISOMETRIC MOVEMENT

Shift back to the flip side of muscle activation for strength. Again, isometric movements mean that your joints aren't moving but your muscles are making force via their contractions. Again, common isometric exercises include wall sits, planks, bridges, and hollow body holds. When you stay in a pose (without joint movement), your muscles are forcefully activated to keep you in balance.

Isometrics may be appropriate for you if low-impact exercise is prescribed, perhaps because of an injury or to a lack of exercise space. A famous golfer named Gary Player used his international flight times to and from his home in South Africa to perform his endured isometric exercises. Isometric exercises build muscle, strength, and bone density. As an extra bonus, they improve cholesterol levels and digestive function—meaning they help lower blood pressure.

Do I prefer one class of muscle activation over another? No. I suggest that you do what you need to do, wherever you find yourself, to maintain and gain functional strength as medicine. I do spend more time in complex isotonic exercise motions, particularly rowing, in which my major joint movements are required. However, I did perform isometric exercises on my long-haul flights as a tourist to and from South Africa and central Europe. While standing watch on the bridge of a ship, I also did isometrics to intermittently work my muscles and to help me stay alert. Are you ready to rethink your body motions and strength in three dimensions? And away you go to build on kinetic counts you read earlier...

PLANES OF BODY MOTION:

Again, your muscles make your skeletal movements possible in these three body planes of motion.

1. SAGITTAL PLANE:

This first axis or plane divides your body into left and right halves, and spatially defines your forward and backward movement. Examples of sagittal plane movements are back squats, bicep curls, walking, running, and climbing stairs (in normal fashion, though climbing stairs sideways and backward are also fine resistance moves too.) Indoor rowing and sculling on the water are another fine examples of sagittal motion. So is stationary or road cycling.

2. FRONTAL PLANE:

This body plane divides your body into front and back halves and defines side-to-side movements. Examples of frontal plane movements are lateral leg and arm raises, jumping jacks, side shuffle and lunges, and side bends.

3. TRANSVERSE PLANE:

Your third plane or axis divides your body into top and bottom halves or defines your rotational or twisting movements. Examples include golf swings, discus throws, plus baseball, tennis and pickle ball swings, and shoulder/hip ball-and-socket movements.[41]

And yes, there are some complex movements that combine muscular efforts in multi-planes. I personally like Turkish get-ups and ninja-warrior moves when you move and work in more than one body plane.

MUSCLE JARGON

Today, we use a common name for a flexed or contracted sarcomere (or skeletal muscle fiber or a little mouse)—namely, a muscle. Yes, in olden days, it was namely "little mice".

Take a big, cleansing breath and acknowledge strange-sounding words and phrases accepted in scientific circles. Please do not think you need a degree in kinesiology or advanced bioscience to appreciate our little mice's biochemical and kinetic functions. There is nothing wrong with vernaculars of *pipes, guns, and wheels* if they are grasped by all parties.

Believe it or not, exact "how's" of muscle contractions to do bodily work are still mysteries among kinesthetic experts. Yet, a few muscle terms should *not* be mysteries for great GenX athletes.

Herein are four muscular terms for a strong GenX:

1. SARCOMERE

A sarcomere is the basic contractile unit of a skeletal muscle fiber. Each sarcomere comprises two main protein filaments—actin and myosin—which are the active structures responsible for muscular contraction.[42] I wish I could share how these intracellular proteins truly get activated and interact. Yet I cannot. Nor can current research experts. **Note:** Sarcopenia is literally a "loss of flesh."

Sarcopenia is progressive with age for normal Joe and Sally Six-Packs. Their generalized loss of skeletal muscle mass and strength begins at about thirty calendar years. A great GenX can delay that unfortunate start. It is strictly correlated with trends toward physical disability, poor quality of life, and death. Risk factors for sarcopenia include age, gender, and level of physical activity.[43] *Do not* be generalized in this risky business. Rather, be a strong outlier of Generation X and stave off the onset of sarcopenia. And when sarcopenia inevitably starts, a great GenX works to slow its progression.

2. MITOCHONDRIA

Mitochondria are membrane-bound cell organelles that generate most of the chemical energy needed to power your biochemical reactions. Chemical energy produced by the thousands of mitochondria per each sarcomere is stored in small organic molecules called adenosine triphosphate (ATP).[44]

3. ATP

ATP (Adenosine triphosphate) is your important "energy currency" in the many mitochondria of each sarcomere. Here is a biochemistry 101 walkthrough: Suppose a cell needs to tap and expend stored energy to accomplish a task. In that case, the ATP molecule splits off one of its three phosphate groups, becoming ADP (*adenosine diphosphate*) plus one free phosphate. Potential energy from bonding that full phosphate molecule is released and made available for kinetic motion. A muscle cell then cyclically stores energy by reattaching a free phosphate molecule to ADP, turning it back into ATP. *Each ATP molecule is just like a rechargeable battery.* When it's fully charged, it's ATP. When it's run down, it's ADP.[45]

4. HYPERTROPHY

Hypertrophy is an increase in muscular size that is gained through tailored exercise of volume, intensity, and tempo. If you want to improve your muscle definition or get "cut," lifting weights is the most common way to increase hypertrophy.[46] With appropriate work, your muscles actually become torn. These micro-tears are inflammations that your body senses and repairs – *if* you aid and abet that repair effort. Assist with proper rest, hydration, and replenishment of complete amino acids to make your fibers a little longer and thicker in a day or two. Note that immediate boosts in muscle size are vascular results from your body's release of nitic oxide. Now, consider these forcing facts about your amazing GenX body.

FORCEFUL KNOWLEDGE

Practical facts that you can appreciate and use as a student of your strong endeavor strong include:

1. Forty percent of an average human's body weight is skeletal muscle.
2. Twenty percent of that skeletal muscle mass is protein. That "fifth" totals only about twelve total pounds of protein mass for the "average" GenX!
3. About half of skeletal muscles' weight is water weight (H_2O). This underscores the uber-importance of hydration for those who lift weights.
4. A male's biceps muscle group weighs only about 1—1.5 pounds.
5. It takes eight to twelve weeks to add measurable muscle size with dedicated work for strength and hypertrophy.
6. Our muscles store about fifteen seconds of intracellular energy to do work before needing replenishment from blood supplies. Then liver glycogen and finally white fat are sequenced to help energize muscle actions. Anaerobic lactate processes also fuel striated muscles for short periods when exertion is too demanding for aerobic energy sources.
7. Human strength is impressive, yet we are humbled by the plyometric power and/or strengths exhibited by nonhuman species (remember Methuselah's Zoo?):
    a. Elephants have more power over their movements than other animals due to their self-contained four-wheel drives.
    b. Ants can lift ten to twenty times their bodyweight—far more than we can!

c. Fleas can high jump up to two feet and broad jump about fifty times their body length! Spoiler alert—the Olympic long jump record is only about five times the victorious athlete's body height.

d. Although the average bite pressure of the human jaw is about 160 pounds per square inch (psi), a Nile crocodile's muscular bite is 5,000 psi!

Unless superheroes Batman and Wonder Woman strut their stuff in real life, we can humbly shift from freakishly strong animals to what is humanly possible for you. Let us think about our sarcomere activation.

Most people can get their nervous systems to activate about *30 percent* of their available muscle fiber in particular muscle groups at one time. Thirty percent. Part of the reason for this batting average is a body's inherent protection or throttling.

FLEX ALERT #16:

Elite athletes are trained to respond with about half (50–60 percent) of their available muscle fibers for a move or activity. Recruiting and activating as many of your little mice as currently possible is a strength imperative.

To be clear, your call to action is to activate and engage more little mice. You will learn how to activate as many fibers as safely possible, with practice.

We flex and extend about *six hundred* different muscles and muscle groups in our bodies to move, achieve balance, and to support our skeletons and internal organs. Provide a precise and actual science-backed number of muscle groups to become a next great champion on *Jeopardy*. Honest, muscle experts still agree to disagree about the exact number of your and my muscle groups. Those brainy folks classify muscles and muscle groups according to their sizes, shapes, actions, and fiber types, which may lead to differences in their scientific counts. *Mox nix.* Whether you have 598 or 602 skeletal muscle groups, *each of* your individual muscle fibers has a mix of two twitchy trigger types, as you'll read next, from our human evolution. Your "twitchiness" is most assuredly different from mine, by the way, as each human athlete is different with a nature- and nurture-blend of fast and slow.

FLEX ALERT #17:

Remember "If you have a body, you are an athlete?" (Bill Bowerman, coach, and Nike® cofounder). This is a perfect time to flex your knowledge of one ancient Greek word. And here is why: "athlete" comes from the Greek word, *athelin*, which means "to compete for a prize." That's what I'm writing about!

With healthy deference to both Coach Bowerman and those competitive Greeks,

- You have an amazing body.
- You compete each day, every day for the prize of your choice.

Ergo, a great GenX is a savvy and worldly athlete who reaches for that worthy prize, that decade as a brass ring on the merry-go-round of life. Back to muscle fiber activations.

If you wonder about my blend of sarcomeres, I am a slow-twitch outlier. Think of me as a Clydesdale work horse rather than an Usain Bolt quarter horse with uber fast-twitch mice. I am an 80 percent slow twitch/20 percent fast twitch kinda athlete. Yup. I am built to last with endured strength and stamina rather than peak power generation. If you ask me to do a plyometric box jump, I'll assuredly underperform the recently retired football standout, J. J. Watt. Challenge me to bike, hike, or row a long distance, and I'm all in. Conversely, speedy muscles of Usain Bolt, the fastest man on earth (as of 2016), are likely 90 percent or higher fast twitch fibers. No work horse duties for you, Usain.

FLEX ALERT #18:

Your age and aging process can change the ratio of slow and fast twitch fibers in your muscles that were wired in your genetic code at birth. As you get along in years, your fast-twitch fibers, whatever their percentage, fade away or become senescent quicker than do slow-twitch fibers.

Make a note: keep working both types of your muscle fibers! Activate and challenge 'em into your ninth decade of life.

IMPORTANT FACTS ABOUT TWITCH

1. Slow-twitch muscle fibers, which are labeled as type I, help you sustain strength and/or stamina activities after their pulsed activation by your central nervous system. At the cellular level, these slow-twitch fibers contain more mitochondria (remember those little powerhouses with ATP for aerobic power generation?) and look darker or redder than their fast-twitch counterparts. Envision the *shaded difference between the thigh meat and breast meat* of a domestic chicken as evidence of denser versus lesser mitochondria in muscles. Why? Type I slow-twitch sarcomeres are better supplied with blood than your second category of muscle fiber.

2. Fast-twitch muscle fibers (Type II) are less dependent on mitochondrial aerobic capacity to generate rapid or "explosive" effort, such as an Olympic lift or an Olympic 100-meter dash.

As a little memory aid, Think of Type 2 fibers as "too fast."

Fast-twitch fibers can be further categorized into Type IIa and Type IIb fiber. Don't get bogged down by that extra twitchy detail for Type II fibers. GenX athletes can do just great by knowing and working these 2 main fiber types—I slow, and II fast. You may be a wee bit curious what slow and fast mean for timing:

- Type II "white or fast twitch" muscles cycle at seventy times per second when pulsed by our nervous system.
- Slow-twitch Type I muscles contract and expand around thirty times each second.

Please make notes that: 1.) relative percentages of each muscle type and top performance capacity change with your calendar age. And 2.) you can continue to develop both muscle fiber types both as you age, though fast-twitch Type II fibers become your bigger challenge. Life happens, so use 'em or lose 'em.

An average athlete may have 50 percent slow-twitch and 50 percent fast-twitch fibers in most skeletal muscles.[47] There is *not* a big difference between men and women in this department. Composition of fast and slow fibers can vary between and among your muscle groups. An uncomfortable formal biopsy with deep core sampling can determine your fiber composition, while making you twitch in discomfort. Shift gears to go both fast and slow in a wonderful compound resistance exercise, the self-explanatory Squat.

DIDDLY SQUAT

Aha and well done. You found this chapter's focus exercise, the squat, which has many variations for velocity, intensity, tempo, and planar focus. *You read and hopefully practiced a bodyweight squat earlier.*

My credentialing body, the National Federation of Professional Trainers recognizes, "(the squat) as one of the toughest and most rewarding exercises you can do to improve flexibility, mobility, and agility. As well as being a leading exercise for your core workout." Highlight those exercise descriptors, *toughest, rewarding, leading,* if you please.

You may choose dumbbells or kettlebells as complements or substitutes for a weighted barbell for your squatting. Consider a "goblet" squat with kettlebell, as illustrated in Figure 4.3 below.

This strength move, with its inherent stability and stretching factors, rightfully has a place in the powerlifting trio of exercises with the deadlift and bench press. Powerful indeed.

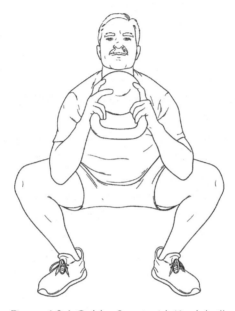

Figure 4.3 A Goblet Squat with Kettlebell

What a marvelous move, this complex, closed-chain squat! Think of the goblet squat (Figure 4.3) as a push movement upward, with your forces driving through the ground connection. Speaking of ground, I often recite *"glutes to ground"* as a client mantra. That is, when their lower bodies and core chains are ready for the near-ground deep range of motion from a standing position, with core muscles fully engaged and glutes activated.

If you don't have a Smith machine or a squat rack, fear not and worry not. You still have squatting alternatives galore.

As mentioned, air squats are a *bueno* bodyweight alternative. Today's knowledge workers should take regular breaks from sitting to rise, then dip their hips to get their heart rates raised with air squats and to offset sleepy gluteal muscles.

Skip squatting at your peril. I jest not.

FLEX ALERT #19:

Dormant butt syndrome (DBS) is an official term that depicts harmful sitting as the new smoking habit. *Oy.*

Avoid DBS now and avoid DBS always.

Consider these steps for a DBS-busting squat movement. Bust away with weights in a front or back or Zercher squat position.

- ✓ Start from a flat-footed standing position, with your toes pointed ahead and feet split at about shoulder width.
- ✓ Engage your core muscles.
- ✓ Bend your knees and push your hips back to lower until your thighs are at least parallel to the floor. Think of this hip hinge as sitting down in a chair.
- ✓ Push through your heels as you mindfully exhale to come back up to your starting position.

Ta da! You just worked major muscle groups— your quads, glutes, lower back, and core—with particular emphasis on those powerful piston quadriceps (which are the longest muscle fibers in your strong body).

PS

Greatness can be yours. You are a squat standout when you can perform a pistol squat (PS) variation of the regular squat to a notable compressed depth. *Put your pointer finger as the barrel, raise your thumb as the pistol hammer; clench your lower three fingers and you have the side view imagery of what a pistol squat looks like.*

Hold this thought: a *unilateral* pistol squat accommodates most of your bodyweight. This is super-solid resistance work even as a bodyweight exercise. Many work up to a free space PS using TRX straps as "training wheels". This is a very good way to address

S.A.I.D. – right? Great ankle mobility and strength (dorsiflexed motion, by the way) are precursors for this strong "PS." You may not become a circus performer with your pistol squats, yet you again prove that it doesn't take much space or equipment to be strong to save. Are there other squat variations? Sure…

Some folks use a weighted vest when they tackle the legendary Memorial Day MURPHY CrossFit WOD which includes *three hundred* squats. Now – that is competing for a prize! You are truly a strong GenX with a completed *Murph* under your belt.

Some folks challenge themselves by squatting to the ups and downs prompted in Moby's song, *Flower*. You'll find that ~ 3 1/2 minutes of squatting to be dynamic and endured effort!

How about squatting with a weighted medicine ball, a ruck sack, or a sandbag?[48] I believe that you get my F.I.T.T. drift. Please study the Squat sequences offered in these images of Figure 4.4:

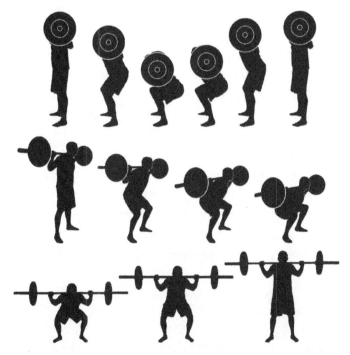

Figure 4.4 A Back Squat Sequence from Three Angles

That cartoon superhero of the 1950s, Mighty Mouse, offers a *save the day* paragon for what strength can and will do you. Yes, even a little mouse can save the day.

STRENGTH MATTERS—MIGHTILY

I don't see *little mice* when I do my upper arm exercises. Hmmm. Perhaps those clever Romans were sipping their foot-stomped Sangiovese when the word musculus popped up? As you consider your own mighty mice or Tecumseh's bundled twigs, you can review why mighty strength mattered for historical figures, rather than TV cartoon characters.

Strength often made the difference between life and death in earlier eras. Legendary Spartans didn't become tough dudes without resistance training with forced muscular adaptation over time. Real-life Scythian horse women were assuredly mighty. Note: Exhibited strength is gender-neutral these days, although ancient Olympic competitors were *omnis viris* (only males.) Today's ninja warriors of both sexes exhibit notable D.E.E.P. strengths. Plus, today's women powerlifters produce about the same lift-to-bodyweight ratios as their male counterparts. You've come a long way, ladies. This is worth rewriting for you: *Strong is your new skinny.*

Strengths in both ancient and modern history need capable connective tissue and joints. Reminder: fascia, cartilage, tendons, ligament, and skeletal bones are parts of our kinetic chains too. Martial art practitioners appreciate these connective tissues and skeletal components of functional strength. Get martial too as you think about your postexercise recovery efforts.

FLEX ALERT #20:

Women tend to recover quicker than men from serious weightlifting sessions. I am envious! Why is this so? Ladies process glucose quicker.

They have more estrogen (duh) and generally have more slow-twitch muscle fibers.

Fast forward your time machine from Athens and Rome to the Scottish Highlands where Braveheart and single-malt Scotch originated. Strongmen in those clans exhibited their "heavy" (or *strang* in Scottish) skills in events like shot put, tug-of-war, caber toss, and hammer throw. These were known as heavy events for a good cause.

HOWDY DOODY

Here is your howdy do reminder: Repetition and repetition regularly shape your success to remain strong to save. Move "right" stuff repeatedly, and you will get toned, become stronger, and be more powerful to cope with adversity. Yes, your "right" stuff comes with delayed muscle soreness (DOMS), and your strong stuff must be fed and rested. Yes, you need to move stuff twice or three times *every* week to down age your fitness or gym years.

Yes! Your body weight and/or special someone will also count as *good* stuff to move by night or day. I like to move it, move it too. What's the plan for you? Your plan will be different than the one used by bodybuilders and elite athletes. Your plan will get you just sore enough to trigger your body's restore and rebuild processes for microtears and inflammation.

Plan and execute your repetitions to be both effective and efficient in your strength workouts. Trust me—the terms reps and sets will become second nature for you.

REPS AND SETS

We call sequential moves *repetitive* for lifting, pulling, pushing, twisting, or carrying actions without a timeout.

1. You can lift, push, pull, twist with, or carry "heavy" for absolute power in a few repetitions (one to six of them).
2. You lift to change your body composition and increase muscle size (aka hypertrophy) with eight to twelve repetitions using medium-weight objects. Note that *medium* is both relative and changing for you in S.A.I.D. ways.
3. And/or you maintain muscle tone and sustain strength with fifteen or more repetitions of relatively light weights.

Power, Hypertrophy, and Toning or maintenance repetitions ... Now, are you *set*?

A set is one group of resisted repetitions performed before you take a break. There is a special repetition term—one repetition as maximum (1RM)—which establishes what a "heavy" weight means for you at this current time. This repetition sets up your tailored, timely activities on a time leg or "period" of your strength journey. You base your chosen weights or resistance for power, hypertrophy, and toning sets as a percentage of 1RM. For example, a 10-repetition set for hypertrophy gains should be about 2/3rds of your current 1RM. Think about that. Someone who has a 300-pound maximal 1RM back squat should plan to use about 200 pounds for hypertrophy sets.

Get comfortable with these strength terms: repetitions(reps), 1RM, sets, PB, and periods. Take your time to gain a working knowledge of these mighty terms. Though ancient Olympians and Scythians may not have known Strength in terms of a Top Ten list, yet you will now:

Your sthenic and formidable top-ten reasons to make each musculus longer and thicker are:

1. Increase bone density from your load bearing exercises. This is ultra-critical for ladies in their middle-ages. *Osteopenia* and *osteoporosis* are as bad for wellness as they sound. Will you permit me to quote *Harvard Health*? "A well-rounded strength training program ... can benefit practically all your bones.

Of particular interest, it targets bones of the hips, spine, and wrists, which, along with the ribs, are the sites most likely to fracture. Also, by enhancing strength and stability, resistance workouts reduce the likelihood of falls, which can lead to fractures."[49] Amen.

2. Delay and/or diminish your loss of skeletal muscle. Avoid at least some of the 3 percent to 8 percent loss of skeletal muscle that bell-curved Billy and Betty suffer each decade as they age. Too bad that we cannot reverse aging factors like this "normal" phenomenon of sarcopenia. Yet, you and I should do our darnedest to defer *loss of flesh* for as long as possible. Nature will eventually overtake your best efforts. That's life. Yet your goal is to get an extra decade before sarcopenia gets an upper hand.

3. Increase lean (vital) mass.

4. Increase resting Metabolic Rate (non-exercise calorie burn!)

5. Reduce unhealthy (white) fat weight – especially around one's midsection.

6. Improve physical performance.

7. Walk faster (a valid longevity factor) and power uphill better on foot or bike.

8. Stay independent longer.

9. Increase insulin sensitivity (an adult diabetes factor that most can address!)

10. Assist in pain management for arthritis and fibromyalgia.

HEY COACH, IS THIS LIST OF MUSCULAR BENEFITS COMPLETE?

No. No list is ever complete as times and people change, and as we learn more about geroprotection. You'll learn more substantive benefits as your turn these *Strong to Save* pages. You'll drill down into these benefits as you get your great work done. Trust me as an uplifting prompt. Speaking of Lifts, please turn your page.

Lift Todd, Tina, and Terry—Lift!

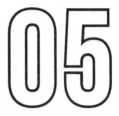

> "Carry a big stick and you will go far."
>
> **—West African proverb**

This African truism was adapted by one of my favorite US presidents, Theodore "Carry a Big Stick" Roosevelt. Here is a quick story to tell about Roosevelt and how far he went...

The Washington Nationals, a major-league baseball team, entertain home crowds with Presidential character races around the ballpark. "Run, Teddy, run" became a game-cry that even was mentioned by presidential candidates Obama and McCain before their 2008 presidential election. You see, the other characters always prevailed over Teddy in hundreds of entertaining races over the baseball seasons. Call it fake news in action, because Teddy won many races as a man of all seasons. Not always, but he was often a victor to be hailed.

- He always competed for the *prize*!

The real Teddy Roosevelt epitomized success and triumph. In his 1899 speech, titled *The Strenuous Life*, Roosevelt preached active lifestyles.

Note: I interpret "man" in this speech as a gender-neutral expression, as we do for "*fireman*" or "*policeman*" these days. Again, strength is gender neutral. So, ladies, you are included in modern *unshrinking* and triumphant ranks when you engage in strenuous lifestyles, too:

"the strenuous life, the life of toil and effort, of labor and strife; ... that highest form of success which comes ... to the man who does not shrink from danger, from hardship, or from bitter toil, and who out of these wins the splendid ultimate triumph."[50]

Our rough rider and warrior president, Teddy, exercised regularly and participated in boxing, horseback riding, hiking, rowing, polo, and tennis. He skinny-dipped in the Potomac River in winter times.[51] Note: Wim Hof, who now advocates cold therapies and champions them in a Wim Hof Method, probably took note of those chilly dips for a strenuous life.

A strenuous lifestyle kept Teddy Roosevelt fit in his middle age. His strength and constitution probably helped him engineer an extended Russo-Japan peace treaty that led to his Nobel Peace Prize award in 1906. That same grit enabled him to finish a campaign speech after being *shot* in the chest. Consider this report: "The horrified audience... on October 14, 1912, gasped as the former president unbuttoned his vest to reveal his bloodstained shirt. It takes more than that to kill a *bull moose*, the wounded candidate assured them."[52]

At the time of his ultimate passage at age sixty in 1919, a witty politician, Thomas R. Marshall, said, "Death had to take Roosevelt sleeping, for if he had been awake, there would have been a fight."[53]

How about that? The bull moose leader and rough rider Teddy was a true die-hard fighter. He survived a perilous expedition along South America's River of Doubt.

His vigorous pursuit of physical and mental strength is a north star for my physical journey. I trust that a great GenX as you will find your guiding star for your strong to save passage.

One additional note: A century ago, sixty years of age was about an average lifespan an American guy. Yet, Roosevelt's strenuous life— from combat service to chest wounds to a malarial river voyage and even wintry skinny-dipping— made him a person in full.

Don't you want to be a person in full too? In ways like the fictional Ulysses, TR could have avoided dangers. That was not in his nature. However, we should remember that it is better to avoid danger – first. Be ready for danger yet be safe.

SAFETY FIRST AND ALWAYS

Be prudent and safe for all your strength and resistance activities. Get your formal approval from a medical professional to engage in TR-like strength activities. *Better safe than sorry* is a platitude for good cause. You may have seen or may have completed a PAR-Q[54] before you worked with a fitness trainer or strength coach like me. I hope so. In my book, and in your *Strong to Save* fit map, you must tune in to your body signals, respect Murphy's Laws, and recognize that you are on a long strenuous journey, the longer the better. Trying to get one more repetition or add too much weight for a "PR" attempt and you may be sorry rather than safe. Both your current strengths and limitations count.

- Know your body and your current capacities to lift, move, and carry objects or move stuff to sweat for *longish* periods. Consider forty-five minutes to an hour as a longish period. Sure, you can work quickly in a time crunch, but forty-five minutes to an hour is a reasonable period to achieve your intended volume, intensity, and tempo of weightlifting for gains. Note: there are occasional shortcuts like a Hotel Room Workout of the Day (WOD) that you read about earlier.
- Get key measurements and know your body type. Consider it essential to start "somewhere", then safely extend and expand what you can and will do. Moderation, Satchel Paige wisely offered, is your pacing advice. Don't chase an impossible dream and suffer injury or experience burnout.
- Don't pass through a door of discomfort to get an extra repetition or move extra tonnage. Discomfort and pain are feedback to which you *must* listen.

Acknowledge that bodily soreness (DOMS) is swell ... well, sort of swell. Post-exercise soreness is a positive sign of your exerted muscles' inflammatory microtears, recovery, and repair cycle. You need these feedback signals. Soreness is a regular acquaintance of yours in the *fortius* world of a great GenX. So, accept its presence (but ensure that your CNS sensation is soreness rather than acute or chronic pain).

Sure, accept the "pain and gain" adage, though I'd rather that you call your postexercise adage "be sore, then restore." Not too much, and not too little. Guys, you won't become an overnight strength-success story. Ladies, becoming Ms. Hercules in a fortnight isn't in the cards you were dealt. Exercise-induced pain or soreness signals *are* telling us something valuable. Even elastic and dynamic superheroes will get sore.

Reminder: You need to build and maintain the size and functional strength of your skeletal muscles or else you will likely become an average Jack or Jill whose muscle mass diminishes with calendar age.

Effective and efficient strength training will help you:

- Strengthen your bones, increase bone density, and reduce risks of osteoporosis.
- Keep your weight in check and increase your metabolism to burn more calories.
- Improve overall quality of life and do everyday chores.
- Decrease your chances of getting or advancing osteoarthritis, obesity, heart disease, depression, and diabetes.
- Improve your thinking skills along with your physical strength.[55]

So, get a grip on heavy things as you develop your formidable physical banking portfolio. Again, note the important link between mind and muscle in that last bullet.

Table 5.1 lists: decent stick, big stick, and great big stick performance measures that TR would assuredly approve, for Todd, Tina, Terry, and for you:

FITNESS OF A DECENT GENX

1. Ably perform activities of daily life as do your generational peers.
2. (a.) Deadlift three-quarters of your body weight (one repetition maximum or 1RM).
   (b.) Show measured grip strength that is normal for your age and gender.
3. Complete a mile walk/run in eleven minutes or less.

GOOD FITNESS OF A GENX

1. Ably perform heavier/longer/harder activities (ADLs) before fatigue, being in the top quarter of your age and gender.
2. (a.) Deadlift more than one times your body weight (1RM).
   b.) Show measured grip strengths of each hand that are strong for your age and gender.
3. Complete a mile walk/run in eight minutes and thirty seconds or less.

GREAT GENX FITNESS

1. Compete in your chosen activities and finish in *the top few (i.e., 5-10) percent* for your age group and gender.
2. (a.) Deadlift more than 1¼ of your body weight (1RM).
   (b.) Demonstrate measured grip strengths for each hand that are very strong for your age and gender.
3. Complete a mile walk/run in seven minutes and forty-five seconds.

Table 5.1: Three Strength Ratings by Ages
Fifty to Sixty (Gender Independent)

Naturally, you may be at a higher or lower performance in a certain activity. If your grip is good instead of great, develop a "biomarker" vice grip to die harder. Note that only the deadlift performance measure in Table 5.1 requires a heavy resistance object. Moving heavy stuff is wonderful medicine, yet bodyweight regimens can work too, as you will read. In fact, one observational study documented that even moderate strength training *lowered death rates by 9%*.

GOOD THINGS COME TO THOSE WHO "WEIGHT"

Todd, Tina, and Terry—do *not* despair if you're temporarily away from heavy metal or other inanimate objects for your resistance exercises. Here is a body case in point: A buddy chair position (the Utkatasana yoga pose in Sanskrit shown in Figure 5.1 below) is a freeform pose to build or sustain your endured core strength without external weights.

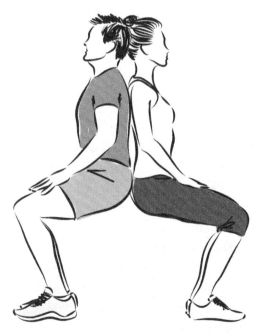

*Figure 5.1 A Couple's "Chair" or Utkatasana
as Bodyweight Exercise*

The classic push-up or press-up is this chapter's focused strength exercise for Todd, Tina, Terry, and for you. This pushing exercise for strength works your muscles and muscle groups of the chest, shoulders, back, and arms. You will use a slew of antagonist muscle groups too.

Notes: if a regular push-up is challenging now, you should start with your hands resting on a wall surface or a small, stable table or a step for your introductory strength motions. My pressing point is to start now, whatever modification is prudent.

Can you get strong with pushups? Absolutely.

Pardon as I cite a very strong and fast athlete who is a tad older than a Gen X birth date, about 18 months older. NFL great, Herschel Walker, directly attributes his strength to *hundreds* of daily pushups in his high school, college, and professional years. I suggest that some of Herschel's running speed is also linked to a very fit chest, shoulder girdle and arms.

Bonus time: you can certainly enjoy push-ups for Sexercise, as detailed in an upcoming chapter. So, here is your protocol for a baseline or "normal" push up.

PUSH UP PROTOCOL

Start in a plank position (prone or face down) with your palms flat on the floor. Place your hands shoulder-width apart, with your shoulders stacked directly above your wrists. Extend your legs with toes bent and properly engage your core.

Then bend your elbows and lower your body to the floor in this negative or eccentric phase. Inhale as you descend.

Sequentially exhale as you push "up" through the palms of your hands, with a plank alignment to straighten your arms in this concentric or positive phase of the move. If you paused at the down position of a push-up, you invested in *an isometric pause*. That's one completed repetition for you.

Note: Once you get accustomed to this "usual" plank pushup starting position, I recommend that you try starting in the down position – with your elbows bent and chest/ knees touching the floor or mat. This "get down" position serves to remind you of the full range of motion you can achieve.

As a guideline, power up concentrically, after (or before) an intentionally slower eccentric or negative phase of a strong push-up. You emphasize your "agonist" or prime mover pectoralis ('pecs') and biceps muscles on the concentric portion of a pushup or press up. Then your "antagonistic" posterior muscle groups – your posterior deltoids, rhomboids, and middle trapezius fibers – work eccentrically for you as you lower in each repetition.

Emphasize eccentric work to become solid as a rock, even if not as chiseled as "the Rock" who advised you to *move it* in your *Strong to Save* introduction. Become an eccentric lover, please. And yes, appreciate the *A-A* opposition of agonist and antagonist muscles. Sometimes it *is* great to be antagonistic. And it is often true that variety can spice up your routine.

VARIETY!

I encourage you to try pushup variants to spice up your bodyweight routines. For instance, try adding a weight vest, for added intensity in any of these pushup variations that follow:

- When you feel ready to challenge some of the smaller regions of your agonist muscles, give a go for "diamond" or "narrow hand" pushups. Narrow means that your palms or fists are closer to your body's midline than in a "normal" shoulder width position. You will sense more emphases on your triceps and anterior delts in a *diamond formation*.
- You can also elevate either your feet or head on a stable weight bench or other elevated platform. I assure you that

you will experience "regional" focus by changing your pushup orientation.

- Or, add a bit of plyometric action to your pushups by clapping your unweighted hands during concentric or eccentric phases.
- To add a stability challenge to a "normal" pushup, unweight one arm and tap that side's hand to the opposite shoulder. Then alternate as you continue your repetitions.
- One of my favorite variants is named after an action hero – Spiderman. As you lower your chest toward the ground (the eccentric phase) of a push up, unweight either leg, and bring your knee toward your distal midback. As you push back up, return your *spidered* leg to the normal plank position.
- Speaking of my favorites, why not try pushups with exercise slides or workout discs? These slides, aka core sliders, challenge your flexibility and ranges of motion as you work your strength. With palms flat on the discs, slide one arm out in any direction as you perform the concentric and eccentric phases of a pushup. Road warriors and travelers: these light and portable discs are great to tuck away in your suitcase or backpack for travel workouts.
- Perhaps you have seen folks do pushups while gripping kettlebell handles as bases. *Just ensure that the kettlebell is big enough to keep from tipping over* - safety first.
  - A variation of this variation is to use a weighted exercise yoga ball to roll between your outstretched hands for alternate pushups.
- For extra credit, you can look for online videos that share the swooping motions of a *Hindu* pushup.
- And try "dive bomber" pushups which add complexity to an already complex exercise. Picture a Battle of Midway dive bomber swooping down before climbing out of the dive.

Use a wide pike position or think of starting in a down dog yoga stance. Swoop your head close to the floor, without letting your hips touch the floor. Then "climb" out of the dive with your head ending forward of your straight arms. Bomb's away.

Notes:

a. Muscle fatigue will likely come earlier when doing these great GenX variations, earlier in your exercised time under tension or in fewer repetitions. For instance, diamond or narrow grip push-ups lead to fatigue "quicker" than normal pushups.

    Why? Smaller muscle regions serve as your focused agonists, so earlier fatigue compared to your "normal" pushups with larger agonists is expected.

b. And finally, to my last push point. For years and years, pushups were *modified* for ladies. Instead of a starting in a prone plank position, it was customary to allow knees to be in contact with the floor. *You've come long ways, ladies.*

    The evolved positional standard for pushups (and coincidentally pull-ups) is now the same for *both* ladies and gentlemen. Credit Title IX, CrossFit®, or other factors for this fine example of equity. As shared in other chapters, gender equity or benchmark parity is present in most matters related to physical banking.

There two other roles of muscles in an exercise to cite for completeness.

A third muscle role is called the synergist or helper muscles. Two synergists for a pushup are your "helper" anterior deltoids and triceps.

The fourth and final role of muscles is called *fixator*.

Primary fixator muscles for pushups are your upper trapezius, your latissimus dorsi ("lats"), your frontal core, and your quadriceps. Finally, the four S-I-T-S muscles that form your shoulder's rotator cuff are also stabilizing fixators for pushups:

- Subscapularis.
- Infraspinatus.
- Teres minor.
- Supraspinatus.

Thanks for taking all this knowledge and process for completing a complex strength move to heart! You will find, if you do not already know, that compound or complex exercises like a pushup or press-up get your left ventricle working pretty hard, increase your respiration rate, and raise your pulse for a period too.

Question: What is a great GenX do while heart rate and respiration recover a bit before your next set?

Answer: Enjoy stretch moves and/or stability poses.

COMPLEMENT STRENGTH EXERCISES WITH STABILITY POSES

Figure 5.2, which illustrates a body hold, also called a boat pose, or, in Sanskrit, a *Navasana* yoga pose, suggests a fine complement for your strengthening push-up or press-up routine.

It is a good practice to complement strength moves with interspersed flexibility and balance moves during your resistance session. This inter-leaving helps you complete time-efficient workouts - with stretch moves and/or stability poses between strength sets. Hold this thought as you envision your hold in a stable boat pose: it is good for Sexercise too.

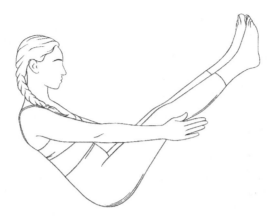

*Figure 5.2: A Boat Pose to Complement
Push-Up Strength Moves*

Protocol: You will start by lying face up (in a *supine* orientation) on a mat with your legs extended and arms straight over your head, keeping them close to your ears. Then contract your abs to press your low back into the ground and lift your legs off the ground. After that motion, lift your shoulders off the ground and keep your head in a neutral position so that you're *not* straining your neck. Your legs and midback should both be off the ground, and you should be in the shape of a banana or "boat," with just your low back and hips balanced on the mat or ground.[56] I underscore how complementary strength sets and stability or flexibility poses, as described here, are *defined* ways to help you down age.

POINT AND COUNTERPOINT...

Point. The overall strength and fitness level of a *decent* GenX gradually declines at about thirty calendar years of age. Then it drops rapidly after those *decent* folks get to their Medicare ages.

Counterpoint: As a great GenX, your habitual exercise and strength regimens *counter* those losses for "normal" folks because you lower your fitness age.[57] As you do this, you make me a happy coach.

Importantly, you increase your health span as a downaged and great GenX.

Characteristics of aging are present in everyone that is *not* a Marvel action hero like Spiderman or a mythical Methuselah. Even a *great* GenX like you can face unfavorable genes, less-than-perfect living environments, and random occurrences that make life with environmental stressors what it is. A critical down-aging component for you, *despite* most misfortunes of life, is your muscle mass. That is, unless you want your visit with Saint Peter to be premature. Another question and answer...

> *Q:Why do even the most sainted priests lift weight?*
> A: Because they enjoy **mass**.

Here are three ways to enjoy your muscle mass to the fullest:

- ✓ Move stuff with volume, intensity, and tempo.
- ✓ Get plenty of restorative rest to let your DOMS-inflamed muscles restore and rebuild stronger.
- ✓ *Eat to live* a strong life with adequate protein and hydration plus those essential and clean micronutrients.

Let's consider a "macro" quantity with a quality all its own, namely complete protein consumption and absorption.

FLEX ALERT #21:

A great GenX should consume ¾ to 1 gram of complete protein per pound of current bodyweight daily to help offset sarcopenia and to help maintain muscle mass. Yes, this protein alert *is* a challenge, yet *you* can meet that challenge.

Example:

A 150-pound lady or gentleman should strive to ingest quality proteins (with all essential amino acids) of *at least* 112 grams per day. This protein should be spaced out as much as possible throughout your day, as a body can only metabolize about 30-35 grams of protein at a time. Three daily meals mean that a great GenX should "slowly" consume at least 30–35 grams per meal setting. If you are an intermittent faster, this compresses to fewer settings, however it is still a doable do. High protein snacks can help you get right amount of daily "clean" protein offsets sarcopenia and helps to repair your exercised muscles (with water and proper sleep).

Yes, it is simple but also quite hard to sustain this commitment. Ass a 150-pounder, think of five daily chicken breasts, or 1½ dozen eggs as dietary equivalents to reach your daily goal of ¾ to 1 gram per pound of bodyweight. Liquid sources and dairy products help me attain this tough protein guideline (that is *above* the Government's recommended daily intake. A great GenX doesn't settle for a minimum—am I correct?)

You might try a trusted protein shake/drink or chocolate milk. Please be diligent to avoid low-quality supplements, and watch out for additives, please. It is only your second-half vitality at stake. Muscle mass and motion are your great GenX vitals. TINA.

Note that your kidneys can handle a much higher level of protein per day than this flex alert amount of ¾ to 1 gram per pound. Remember that this goal is true for both women and men. How you manage this mandate is your personal choice. More protein equates to a *higher* metabolic rate; your amazing body's furnace works a bit harder to process and absorb those essential amino acids than it does for either fats or carbohydrates. That is biochemistry 201. As the Rolling Stones sang...

START ME UP

It is never, never, never too late to start your *Strong to Save* regimen, despite any lifestyle, physical condition or dietary challenges that confront you. Second halves often have surprises, so it is good to expect the unexpected.

Here are three starters that also serve as finishers:

- The earlier you push yourself to be strong, the easier it will be to achieve a long health span as your ROI.
- Proper fueling is a prerequisite to stay Strong to Save.
- As Peter Drucker advised, good plans degenerate into hard work.

An Olympic champion, Michael Brake, told me that I better train as if I was #2 or in second place. He also advised me to be a student of my endeavor and to surround myself with resources.

Take note, please, as this is great tutorial advice for you. You are not alone unless you choose to be. Get a longer healthspan by getting smarter about your functional strengths and how you must nurture them. Get older later and die harder by following the guidance of great practitioners. And find good folks to be your mentors or sounding boards.

Never think that you are lifting with one hand tied behind your back. Be studious and resourceful to gain strength, like yesteryear's stoics and like modern Olympic champs.

Invaluable resources for you abound in print and in digital formats. Please contact me if you think you are *knowledge-poor* as a student of strength. Remember: it is vitally important to be a student of your endeavor. Learn from others and get goin' now – *not* tomorrow or next month - **now**.

One of many reliable resistance and strength resources that I rely upon is called *Breaking Muscle* (breakingmuscle.com). It is *not* happenstance that Breaking Muscle staff members challenge you to be the smartest person in the gym, wherever that workout spot is for you.

Similarly, you can consult the NFPT (my credentialing organization), the ACE,[58] and Livestrong.[59] CRAAP-tested resources stand out with their authentic and effective exercise and health-related content.

As my caveat, be resourceful yet also *skeptical.* Our "online" information age can seduce you with *un*validated figures and too-good-to-be-true claims from *less* reputable sites than those I just cited.

Trust but verify as Ronald Reagan, a strong-for-his-age leader, once reminded us. That is wise counsel for you. Verify how your ten-million-dollar corpus is invested and how it banks your strengths for down aging.

More *validated* knowledge to help *you* become a strong student is next.

PLAN YOUR EXECUTION.

A timed exercise design protocol is called *periodization.* You will experience three timed exercise cycles in your bespoke periodization:

a. A *micro cycle* is the training period designed for you that lasts from one to four weeks, focusing on daily or weekly training variations.

b. Your *mesocycle* is a "mid" training period of two weeks to four months, and it focuses on your progressive goal(s) for optimized performance.

c. And your *macrocycle* includes your long-range training plan from six months up to several years. This long-haul protocol is your framework to achieve optimal performance in a future event, like the Olympics are for elite athletes.

These 3 periodic timeframes for cycles are generalized rather than specific.

If undulation and nonlinear processes intrigue you, then ask your trainer or do your own research about these *special* periodizations. That mentioned, I've never done undulating periods of strength work, and I think I turned out fine.

Formalize a plan of attack, then move stuff, whatever workout cycle you find yourself in. Don't make things more difficult than you are willing to sustain. Going *open kimono* can be easy or hard, it is up to you.

NEKKID

Be open to reflect on real, no-kidding, *deep-down* goals for your strength and health span. Remember that you are a unique athlete to go your own way in life. Remember that impeccable performances usually arise from impeccable bodies. Aleks Salkin, aka the "Hebrew Hammer", first states,

"You want to feel better, get stronger, and build some more internal confidence in your abilities."

Wait, wait… Aleks then challenges you with your next sixty-four-thousand-dollar question and answer:

> Q: *But what do you* really *want deep down?*
> A: Whether a lad or a lass, it's to look good *nekkid.*"

Think about this unclothed fundamental of human nature. Lean, strong bodies do *not* need kimonos, although Aleks may need a spell checker…

THE AESTHETICS PYRAMID

Good and great aesthetics help you *stand out* from most others in your generation. Sturdy, lean, supple, and strong are attractive qualifiers for your physical bank's cornerstone.

With cycles (periodizations) for strength work in mind, let's look at pyramids. These structures are *not* the Incan or Egyptians structures of ancient periods, although those wonders certainly have shown long "macrocycles."

You will preplan and then move stuff in progressive upward phases. You might compare these phases to a pyramid's upward layers—from foundation to penthouse.

✓ The foundation is called stabilization,
✓ the middle layer of the pyramid promotes your muscular size (hypertrophy) and dynamic strength, and
✓ the penthouse phase is for your exhibited peak power.

Foundation: fundamental stabilization is your pyramid's base layer for that entire second half of your life.

Bodily stabilization is your preventative and planned maintenance for an amazing health span. This sturdy maintenance phase assures stability for your muscles, skeletal joints, and connective tissues. Foundational strength movement should factor *imbalanced* work on one body side, a Bosu ball, or on a yoga pad to challenge your stabilizing support muscles and fixators. Remember that S.A.I.D. starts at this foundational layer for strength.

Your foundational focus is on *endured* strength and injury prevention. Generate exercise-induced sweat to ramp up those favorable cytokine message streams. This foundational layer can be a "macro" periodization to increase and maintain your flexible ranges of motion (ROM) too. Of course, quality nutrients and sleep are cast in this fundamental pyramid layer.

Main Floor: your middle pyramidal layer is a hypertrophy and strength (H & S) or "meso" phase to maintain and grow your skeletal muscles (sarcomeres). Your H & S efforts fend off dreaded sarcopenia which hits *"indecent"* or *decent* GenX folks at about age thirty.

How and why? Focused efforts in this mesocycle increase your muscle fiber size and capacity. A nominal H & S period lasts ~ two to three months to achieve specific size and strength gains.

Think of using your *dynamic* strength efforts with relatively "heavy" weights or resistance in this H & S *meso* periodization. And yes, think of delayed onset of muscle soreness (DOMS) when your volume, intensity, and tempo of H&S workouts increase. You know that a "clean" diet and restorative rest are uber-important for your H & S gains, right?

Again, the H & S focus is on adequate volume and disciplined tempos of muscular motions for eight to twelve weeks to achieve noticeable gains and progressive "ROI."

Tip-top Shape: then, you can scaffold to the penthouse of your personal strength pyramid. Your tip-top layer and periodization is when and where *explosive* and *peak* performance can safely be achieved.

You previously built a stable and flexible base to accommodate specific and intense work.

Then, you built up your muscle size and boosted your dynamic strength in H&S.

Now you can celebrate your progressive personal records at a sequenced power peak, like a Bull Moose President or like a Scythian female warrior.

However, progress is never linear over time. In my flat-out candor, even a rough rider or capable Scythian horsewoman will reach a hiatus, a plateau, or a flattop at some points in their macrocycles. That is, on the level.

LA MESA

Fact: You will reach predictable, yet frustrating performance plateaus or mesas at certain points in your strength journey. These mesas or plateaus are recurring *de facto* things.

Why? When you formulate and carry out a physical routine, your body successfully adjusts to the demands of those workout sequences over time. As you reach those mesas or plateaus of your periodizations, you might feel unmotivated, bored, or waver in your commitment.

- Your great GenX mission is to adapt, overcome, and succeed with a game plan to get past la mesa and to resume your ascent.

You see, when strength (or stamina) exercises become more comfortable over a cycle, their training effects *decrease.* Or perhaps you overtrained a bit, or perhaps it is part of the circle of demands of life. Whichever factor was a root cause, you experience a *flattened* performance period.

This flat phase will hopefully be short in duration (weeks) and hopefully will *not* occur close to an upcoming competitive event of yours. Peaking too soon or too late can indeed happen. I am living proof of plateaus and missed peaks in my athletic career. *Ship happens,* says this navy veteran. So, like Murphy, try to avoid "flats" at the worst possible times in your journey. Would you challenge what martial-arts legend, Bruce Lee, once offered?

There are no limits.

There are only plateaus, and you must not stay there for too long. Move on smartly to stretch for new limits. I share some smarty-pant approaches that work to renew your ascents.

ADAPT AND OVERCOME

- Vary your workout routine. Remember the CrossFit philosophy of a highly variable workout for each day? Change things up to stay motivated, keep your approach fresh, and be more effective in building muscles. Remember spice is nice.
- Mix up the sequence of your exercises.
- Drop exercises you have outgrown or that have become redundant. Examine your present regimen with a critical eye and replace out-of-date workouts with ones that are more appropriate for your current fitness level.
- Take a break! Sometimes, it's best to take your foot off the accelerator and sniff the begonias along your roadway. But do not coast for too long, just time enough, as you will learn.
- Tweak or rebalance your diet to pack in more clean nutrients.
- Nap and sleep more, like champions do.

FLEX ALERT #22:

You reach your peak performances *only once or twice* a year. That is twin-peaks physiology without exception.

Twice is nice! This could mean a total of eighty or more performance peaks to come in your healthspan.

It also means that you should *not* strive for, nor can you achieve personal bests in every strength session. So, plan your periodization around key dates (perhaps a decade birthday), or a competition once or twice a year, every year, for the balance of your healthspan. Stay in the arena as Teddy Roosevelt wrote.

Don't ignore symptoms of fatigue, low energy levels, insomnia, and libido loss when you are on a plateau. Do consider a rest break and change the focus of your training cycle's volume, intensity, or tempo. Are you locked on?

LOCKED ON AND TRACKING

This tactical phrase, locked on and tracking, was one I used in my Navy days. We needed to know that our shipboard *sense and respond* systems were working as they should for successful encounters or engagements. Sure, my sense and respond efforts were not all that different than those of which William Whiting wrote in the 19th century.

- Sense your need for proper warm-up and cool-down efforts. These are vital parts of your sense and respond efforts for your exercise induced stress and DOMS, and proper stretching will help you regain your ascent.

Never neglect either your dynamic warm-ups or static cool-down periods. *Nunca. Conglai bu.*

Well, you could skip your warm-up stretches against my advice, but that avoidance could lead to lock *down* instead of lock *on*! This is your tactical call to make.

Proper preparation of your mind and body for sweat with resistance work should be a flash of the obvious. Highlight or dog-ear this:

- your dynamic pre-workout stretches and static après moves need *only* take five to ten minutes each to complete.

Excuses for skipping pre- and après stretching simply do not fly. Make the time, please.

Dynamic warm-ups, either activity-specific or general in nature, prepare your body for the work to come. You'll elevate your body temperature and increase blood flow to your muscles and connective tissues. Limbering up sore muscles from DOMS and preventing injury are valuable reasons to dynamically stretch. Note: you want to engage and prepare the muscle groups and body regions that are used in your sporting event or activity. Whether specific or general, I encourage you to "move it, move it" in all three body planes.

In my case, I limber up with wall, floor, and door stretches, and then I progress to doing actual rowing motions on an indoor rower before we launch a crew shell for practice.

Keep in mind that the wall, floor, and door are true pals for your effective stretches, whatever are your intended activities or exercises.

APRÈS

Slow, static stretches of about twenty to thirty seconds help your body and mind shift gears from its "fight and flight" sympathetic mode after your work is done. Your exercise-induced stress will lessen as you mindfully align your mind and body anticipate a recovery and prepare for your important "rest and digest" phase. Note: A reasonably high Heart Rate Variability (HRV) measure from a fitness device is a fine way to assess how *rest and digest* is faring against the cortisol-driven *flight or fight* half of your neuromuscular system.

Breathe mindfully and stretch statically - as soon as you can - after you complete your heavy work. Do these stretches before your core body temperature cools down.

Three key takeaways for these sustained holds après stretches:

- Don't bounce. Your endured, low-load approach allows a slow time release and a lengthening of your muscles and connective tissues.
- Breathe deeply and mindfully to sink as deeply as comfortable into a static yoga position like a pigeon pose, a frog pose, or into a full hurdler's stretch. *Call me if you can't find protocols for these super stretches, either online or in the library.*
- Listen to your body and stop static stretching if discomfort or pain appears. Pain is a useful feedback signal, so ignore that signal at your own peril, so to speak.

BEFORE

Warm up and perform dynamic stretches - before your workouts - sequentially from your smallest to largest muscle groups. Recall that your resistance work has the *opposite* protocol, which is to challenge your biggest muscles first, and then proceed to smaller musculus or little mice. Yes, even cows use a similar sequence protocol.

> Q: Do you know why even cows have leg-day workouts?
> A: Because they need to look out for their *calves*.

REAR GUARD

Now, jump to your rump—or your gluteal muscles—for good reasons.[60] Work your glutes ardently to avoid gluteal *dysfunction* that can cascade to other kinetic chain issues if it is not identified and corrected. Gluteal muscles, the largest in your body by weight, are, in Old English, "protuberances which form the rump." Each protuberance may weigh up to about five pounds, which is an enabler for an athlete's explosive power in events like sprinting or Olympic weight lifts.

And now for the great news…You will perform great in strength, stamina, stability, and stretching regimens when your gluteal muscles are activated and strong. Two community benchmarks for relative gluteal strength are:

- A great GenX is *glute-strong* by properly performing thirty or more donkey kicks with each bent leg from a quadruped (bear crawl) stance.
- A GenX is also *glute-strong* by performing a 1RM *hip thrust* with over 185 pounds for women and over 250 pounds for men loaded across their hips.

Even if you're more interested in the aesthetics of gluteal shape than strength, please understand this:

- Mindful and proper gluteal activation yields functional strength of this *powerhouse* muscle group. This is your sure path to muscle-up performance. Great!

IFS, ANDS, AND BUTTS

Three gluteal muscles are formed by eight skeletal muscle sections in each of your buttocks. Their contractions and linkages to the pelvis and femur bones enable or support *most* human motions from our armpits to our knees. For completeness, we should also consider two regional muscles:

- the piriformis, which can become a common source of backside or leg pain, and
- the psoas, which you read earlier, can create hip flexor dominance that weakens your desired gluteal contractions to move and do work.

Your author speaks with personal experience about sciatica and piriformis syndrome,[2] also known as *deep gluteal symptom*. These neuromuscular disorders occur when a long sciatic nerve is irritated by the proximate and deep piriformis muscle in either buttock. As our National Institute of Health advises, piriformis syndrome is quite common (with *three million* cases reported annually). This syndrome may last months to become a *chronic pain in the arse*, even with medical care or physical therapy. Yet, keep the faith as you can work that discomfort or pain out with balanced and conscientious remedial efforts. Or better yet *preemptively* address these sources of dysfunction.

SOURCES OF GLUTEAL DYSFUNCTION

Three ways that gluteal dysfunction may arise are *seated* in:

- **Lifestyle.** You may be inactive or spend an inordinate time in a sitting position, thereby lengthening and weakening the muscles.
- **Irritation.** You may experience pain because of an irritated sciatic nerve that passes through each gluteal region. This irritation is usually one-sided or unilateral.
- **Tendinitis.** Chronic sitting, excessive cardio exercise (like running) and inadequate strength training can create tendon inflammation. As tendinitis starts, inflamed gluteal muscles are called on to perform repetitive actions for which the tendons are not equipped. The resultant tendinopathy can shut down muscle contractions, to effectively inhibit recruitment of your glutes.
  - ○ When our gluteal actions are *inhibited*, they may "forget" their main purpose of supporting the pelvis and keeping the lumbo pelvic hip complex (or LPHC) in proper alignment.

The medical term for this muscular forgetfulness triggered by tendinitis is *gluteus medius tendinopathy* (GT). Many professional trainers may recognize these other synonyms for GT—namely gluteal amnesia, and/or dormant butt syndrome or DBS.

One's *forgotten* and underappreciated glutes may become a *major* cause of lateral hip pains. Strength and stretching regimens are how a great GenX will preemptively avert hip and LPHC pains or remediate such "core" pains that do arise.

Fact: GT tendinopathy is the *most common* tendinopathy in our lower bodies. Ouch. Women are impacted by GT or DBS more than men in their activities of daily and nightly life.

One NIH report states that *25 percent* of women over age fifty can be affected by this "GT" tendinitis between their *gluteus medius* and hips.[61]

I have trouble spelling *sacroiliac*, and I am troubled if a client has painful problems around her or his sacroiliac (SI) joint. Another drumroll, please: many SI-joint problems can be overcome with proper strength and stretching regimes.

COUNTERACTIONS

First, the simple, yet hard approach to counteract a GT or a DBS of a sedentary lifestyle is to *break up* long periods of sitting. Stretch and movement breaks also limit your chances to get a potentially deadly deep vein thrombosis (DVT). I speak from an author's seated experience that gluteal problems and/or syndromes can become both a hassle and hindrance. *Don't* let your gluteal muscles and/or *piriformis* hassle or hinder you!

PIRI-WHAT?

Deeply situated in each of your *buns* is a pear-shaped lateral muscle that may become a real pain. Its location to your sciatic nerves on each side, plus its roles in both hip adduction and abduction can lead to misalignment and inflammation. Ouch. So, lets align the importance of gluteals with repeat piri- performances.

THREE-PEAT

Your *glutes* have three muscles in each buttock:

1. GLUTEUS MAXIMUS:

This largest gluteal muscle is the one that gives the shape to your butt. This muscle is responsible for keeping us upright when sitting or standing.

2. GLUTEUS MEDIUS:

This muscle is between *maximus* and *minimus*, as the name suggests. This muscle is responsible for rotating your leg and stabilizing your pelvis.

3. GLUTEUS MINIMUS:

As this smallest of the three and the innermost gluteal muscle the *minimus* helps rotate your lower limbs and keep the pelvis stable while moving.

I may sense gluteal discomfort or pain after my power deadlifts, for example. Or perhaps as importantly, I can experience DBS after I sit for more than fifteen minutes without changing position. This image (Figure 5.3) suggests what can happen when *excess* sitting becomes *evil* for someone:

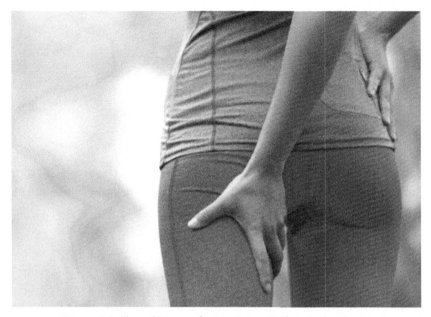

Figure 5.3 Gluteal Discomfort or Pain—Piriformis Syndrome

If you sense a painful *piriformis syndrome* (as seen in Figure 5.3), then respond to strengthen and align your piriformis in yoga positions, or use ranges of motion in 3 body planes to correct your loss of internal hip rotation.

BUTT WHAT?

To counteract or hopefully to avoid that GT or DBS, please activate, stabilize, and exercise your booty with isolation exercises and stretches almost every day.

- Perform yoga moves or *asanas* to promote your glute activation and strengthen those core fibers as you breathe for a mind-muscle connection.
- Improve your hip stability for gluteal strength.

- Prudently pick, choose, then use some of sixteen exercises for your *gluteus maximus* (Gmax) in each buttock.[62] Yup, sixteen.

Figure 5.4 illustrates a pose (called the "figure four") that unlocks your hips and helps avoid a future pain in the butt!

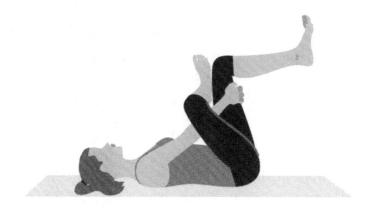

Figure 5.4 A "Figure Four" Stretch to Unlock Your Hips

I am a proponent of two *animal* asanas—the pigeon pose and the frog pose—to work my hips and to gain competitive advantage. Believe it or not, complex exercises like back squats, lunges, and deadweight lifts *don't* optimally develop one's gluteal muscle groups. Thus, isolation moves are needed.

Granted, the glutes are kinetically involved in these exercises, but *if* your quads and/or hamstrings are dominant, and if glutes are "sleepy" their recruitment is diminished as is physical performance. I advocate that you *focus* on isolation exercises to get your buns of steel activated, stabilized, and exercised.

Just think of your activities of daily life and overall strength moves that require those glutes and *piri-what* muscles. If you need a glutes expert to validate these challenges, look up Bret Contreras, PhD. as a highly respected "glute guy."

PINCH-TOUCH-OPPOSE-WORK

These four tactile takeaways should help you overcome gluteal inhibition to improve your performance in daily and nightly activity.

- "Pinch your glutes" is a call to action (or CTA) that cues glute power for nearly every exercise that hinges your LPHC or rotates a hip. Compress or pinch 'em and power on.
- Touch a gluteal region during a core exercise to stimulate the mind-muscle connection. For example, while doing a side scissor kick on the floor, place your upper hand on your buns' side to feel and celebrate the medial work of a gluteal.
- Activate your glutes by working opposing muscles like the psoas (for your glute bridge) and hamstrings (for your Good morning hip hinges).
- Work your glutes in all three body planes—transverse, frontal, and sagittal. And please work 'em in 3D daily.

FLEX ALERT #23:

It is an absolute must do, or imperative to *activate* and strengthen your glutes for a longer and better health span. As songstress Shakira advised, hips don't lie. So don't let sleeping or dormant butts lie either.

EUREKA! THE LUNGE

You've now reached this chapter's focus strength move for Todd, Tina, and Terry: namely the Lunge. Yes, great lunges come in many fun variations, like side, rear, and walking lunges. If you think I mistyped *many* variations, *Women's Health Magazine* listed <u>forty-three</u> variations of your classic strength, stability, and stretching move.

The lady in Figure 5.5 is using a resistance band to optimize her forward lunge workout at a gym. However, you do not need to go to a gym or buy a "booty band" to benefit from lunges. Your lunges only require only a stride's floor length to move, or even a prison cell if you had bad luck and wear orange workout gear. Find a suitable stride space and then slowly and safely lunge away.

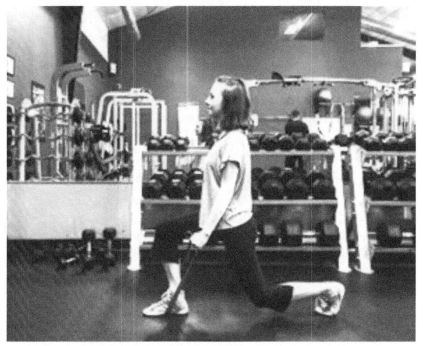

Figure 5.5: A Forward Lunge with Resistance Band

You can emphasize lunge motions in all three body planes by adding a torso twist and box sequence to your important lunges.

Deliberate, *not* uncontrolled, lunges mimic the act of reaching forward to pick something up off the floor. In short, you leave one foot back to work your trailing quadriceps and move one forward as in to step and reach for stretching and stability gains. As the NFPT reminds us:

"When properly executed, lunges effectively develop and empower your lower body quadriceps, calves, hamstrings, and glutes, while raising your heart rate."

Never pass up the chance for a little "cardio" as you work on your dynamic or endured strength. By working one leg at a time unilaterally, your properly executed lunge requires balance, agility, and, in some cases, significantly more leg strength than other leg exercises. Take the plunge with a Lunge.

Choose a correct lunge load (if weighted, not bodyweight), execution speed, and movement pattern based on your current abilities and confidence. If you are ready now as a great GenX, go lunge or go home (I *am* jesting). Engage in lunges after mastering squat or leg press motions to ensure that you provide safe support of your bodyweight (or more) over an extended gait or stride baseline.

Learn to love lunges and their variations. They help you perform longer and better. Longer and better can be by day or night, in a gym box or bedroom.

Kindly hold on to this quote as you begin your next chapter, Sexercise as GenXercise, and throughout your long and productive life.

Before turning your page, consider the strong habit of a hobbit author.

The Oak that is strong does not wither.
—JRR Tolkien, author

Sexercise™ as GenXercise

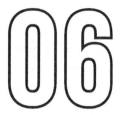

> "Frequency of sex has been linked to *greater* mental and physical health."
>
> **—T. Cabeza de Baca, research scientist**

Great for greater news! As de Baca shared from his team's credible research, *getting it on* means healthier and happier health spans. Period.

INTIMACY IS HEALTHY.

Living large and loving well may include congress, and I am *not* writing about one's elected officials. Having "congress" is healthy for a slew of mental and physical reasons. Even the AARP cites important reasons to get intimate in midlife and later. Hold that image! The world's largest lobbying organization promotes sex in encore years. Now, that is a promotional plug to pursue.

Go ahead and promote that Marvin Gaye classic "Get It On." Or use *Marvin Gaye* as a verb, as Charlie Puth and Meghan Trainor did in their 2017 release, "Let's Marvin Gaye and get it on …" Let's move on to an intercourse of chemistry and animal spirits.

Your intimate chemistry is at work both by night and by day when you are a great GenX. It is working to sense and respond via little compounds, or hormones. As one example, your sensing chemistry can stimulate the responsive hugging hormone, oxytocin. As a plus side in your modern life, Healthline.com authors state that you do *not* need to be in congress to get that happy sense-and-respond chemistry a goin' for your pleasure. In other words, "You don't have to get down to get your oxytocin up."

Yes! Episodic hugs of about twenty seconds can offset stressing cortisone levels. Pretty cool, right?

As your pleasure goes up, your stress goes down. Note: Two other hormones also move in opposite directions to cortisol levels in our biochemistry. Serotonin and dopamine are among the tens of chemical messengers that favorably relate to your very own pleasure palace:

- Serotonin, which is mostly manufactured in your gut, is an antidepressant that responds to happy events.
- Dopamine, as a key *think-and-play* neurotransmitter, is a driver for your reward and motivation.

Now, back to time passages for your hugging hormone. Why did I write "about twenty seconds?"

Men from Mars may need to hug for about thirty seconds to generate their innate oxytocin flows.

Lucky ladies from Venus may need only about ten seconds to gain a similar flow of their amorous hugging hormones. *Viva la difference.* I made an average calculation of (30+10/2) to come up with 20 seconds. However, there is absolutely *nothing* average about a great hug.

Fact: we are wired to frolic and reap neurochemical rewards!

Now I rhetorically ask, is "too much of a good thing truly wonderful?" The answer depends on which half of your "4F" nervous system is dominant on a given day or night. Is it the fight or flight half, or is it (hopefully) your feed and frolic half?

GAME-NIGHT READY?

Guys, rather than making your pipes pop and forearms look like interstate roadmaps before congress is in session, try gentle yoga. Right, choose yoga over bench presses to arrive as ready to play on game night. I highlight that yoga serves as gentle foreplay by stimulating blood flow."[63]

NOT QUITE READY?

An athlete who is training very hard, or perhaps who is riding to excess on those uncomfortable racing bicycle seats, may need more "rest and restore" time before frolicking at will.

Exercise is very good for all of us, *to a point*. Your voluntary (parasympathetic) nerves are relegated to the sympathetic fight and flee subsystem when you train too hard, too fast, or too long. Consider elite Tour de France riders who don't have much time for yoga or a dalliance. Their "overtrained" high-performance racing mandates both mega nutrition and sleeping solo to counter bodily inflammation and to maximize restorative sleep before a next day's ascent.

I digress to recommend the 2017 streaming documentary, *ICARUS*, which begins with cycling steroids and ends with Vladimir Putin's enemy number one hiding in our witness protection program. Kudos to reporter Bryan Folger and to Russia's doping genius, Grigory Rodchenkov, for their exposure of how Russia beat the (PEDs) performance-enhancing-drugs monitoring system. I betcha you sense both my aversion to PEDs and my promotion of au naturel hacks for sexercise and GenXercise. Back to your restoration hardware ...

We can skip the Tour de France's elite yellow jersey. Rather, consider your environmental stressors in modern life. Your professional or personal stresses boost cortisol, for instance. Hormonal changes—from ladies' menopause and even gentlemen's andropause deficiencies or *manopause*—can adversely affect intimacy. To pile on, I offer a midlife image (See Figure 6.1.) for both ladies and gentlemen for what is no laughing matter.

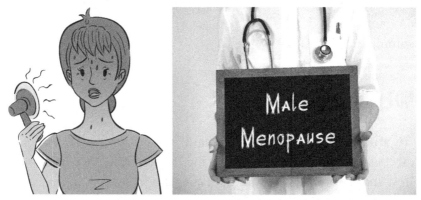

Figure 6.1: Menopause and Manopause (aka Androgen Deficiency in Aging Males (ADAM))

MOOD MATTERS

One or more stressors can supplant your desire and lower blood flows to certain central body regions. As a GenX, you don't like fake news or long cuts.

Disclosure: I did not understudy for Doctors Masters and Johnson. I am neither Doctor Ruth nor Doctor Phil. I didn't co-found the Institute for Research in Sex, Gender, and Reproduction with Dr. Alfred Kinsey. Neither am I that Indian philosopher and author of legend, Vatsyayana Mallanga.

Now this last-mentioned author can help one get in the mood. Vatsyayana wrote a "pleasure bible" named the *Kamasutra*. Now, with all disclosures made, let's get to Sexercise as *very* good GenXercise with *mutual* pleasure and with holds that do matter.

HODL

The *Kamasutra* describes liberating and hold-on-for-dear life (HODL) positions like the colloquial lift, lotus, face-off, G-whiz, pretzel dip, and magic mountain. Checklists or visual training aids for these provocative positions are not provided herein. They are left to your imagination or assigned to your partner and you for tonight's homework.

As is the case for William Shakespeare's amazing body of work, many folks think that the *Kamasutra* was authored by multiple men. My point is:

Whether or not good ol' Vatsyayana was a lone literary ranger, he believed that delightful deeds should promote pleasure for *both* sexes rather than merely to serve for perfunctory procreation.

Hold on for dear life. HODL with that duality for a few moments... he asserted that pleasure and procreation should coexist. Lovely.

COMING TO TERMS

Translating words of mutual pleasures from Sanskrit to the King's English can be hard for us who hardly know a *lingam* from a *yoni*.

Yet one explorer named Richard Burton was able to get that translation done with a colleague named Foster Arbuthnot in 1883. Imagine the buzz that their translation caused back home in prudish Victorian society. Today, there is nothing wrong in coming to terms with steamy Sanskrit writings, the urban dictionary, or in the new King's language. Figure 6.2 is your foreplay for this very pleasurable type of GenXercise.

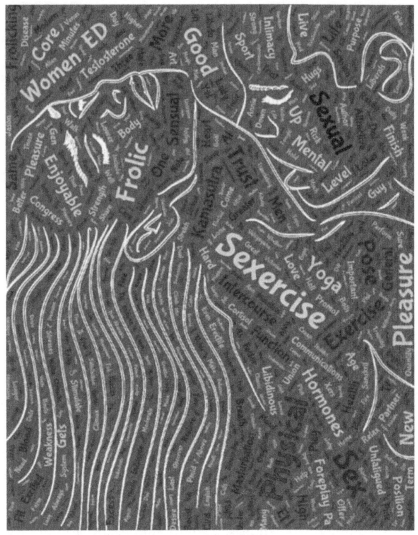

Figure 6.2 Sexercise™ as GenExercise.

I'm not sharing anything new about sexy tips or frolicking. After all, Adam and Eve had healthy appetites and temptations of the flesh too. Sex and exercises that aid and abet erotic muscles and pleasure points are primal elements of our heritage and biochemistry. Let's acknowledge those *trysty* testaments, then ask … *Who* do we thank for the term *Sexercise™*?

A clever guy named Jason is who.

THANK JASON

Let us begin with words of that clever Jason Rosell, who created Caliente Fitness in New York City. His novel branding promotes "a little burn and plenty of *blush*" to help consenting adults "gain longevity on the dance floor or in the bedroom."

Jason made his fitness business by marketing Sexercise™ moves like the anaconda, booty bops, and caliente squats.

Here is Jason's proof positive: A lucky female reporter from the *NY Daily News* learned the anaconda move with Jason as her sexercise trainer. "Rosell instructed me to *anaconda* my legs around him and crunch my abs to pull him deeper and deeper toward me … That move empowers women who want to take control in the missionary position."[64]

Deeper, empowered women, and a big snake. These words create quite a mental image. Hold on girls and guys, do not be a *yold* in a Texan's all-hat, no-cattle sense. Why? This *yold's* response to his amorous bride paints many words:

> Wife: "Honey, let's go upstairs and make love."
> Husband: "Darling, I cannot do both."

And, ladies, you can be a cowgirl, with or without your hat. What are the some of the many moderating benefits of sexual conduct for ladies and gentlemen?

SEX IS BETTER THAN RAKING LEAVES

Researchers at Harvard University studied the physiological effects of sex on males. Ladies – ditto for you…just type keywords" women's sexual health" in your browser to find Harvard Medical School articles about pleasure, and probabilities that sexercise and sex after age fifty *can be* as nice as it was when you were twenty. Just sayin.' Back to you guys…

"Men seem to spend more energy thinking and talking about sex than on the act itself. During sexual intercourse, a man's heart rate rarely gets above 130 beats a minute, and his systolic blood pressure (the higher number, recorded when the heart is pumping blood) nearly always stays under 170 mmHg. All in all, your average sexual activity ranks as *mild to moderate* in terms of exercise intensity ... that is about the same as doing the foxtrot, raking leaves, or playing ping pong. Sex burns *about* **five calories a minute**; that's four more than a man uses watching TV, but it's about the same as walking the course to play golf. If a man can walk up two or three flights of stairs without difficulty, he should be in shape for sex."[65]

Hmmm. I suggest that a great GenX can take many flights of stairs two or three at a time. Guys, please extrapolate the difference of "shape for sex" and the need for stamina on your own.

Consider credible statistics for her "big O." First, ladies need and appreciate longer foreplay than most guys in heterosexual intimacy. Then, ladies may need 12-13 minutes of anaconda play to vaginally climax. You'll come to a true mismatch in climax timing in a few paragraphs. HODL.

Remember Jack LaLanne, the early fitness guru I mentioned in chapter 1? I assure you that he *wanted you* to watch him on TV in the 1960s and 1970s. Ladies, Jack was a pioneering advocate of fit ectomorphic and mesomorphic women. And I assure you that he wanted your buy-in that sex is *unequivocally good* exercise. Well, not as a big calorie burner exercise, but a good-and-pleasurable exercise, nonetheless. Read on for pearls from this early fitness promoter.

LaLanne's candid 1984 interview for *Playboy Magazine* included these four pleasure pearls:

1. We're sensuous creatures.
2. Sex is the greatest driving force on this planet.
3. Why are we living if we can't have a little fun?
4. Sex is giving.

That sounds very much like *Kamasutra* principles of mutual pleasure to me. Let's look at a clever and innovative "buddy" exercise in the spirit of giving. An Aussie observation from *GQ Australia* was, "If you need any more libido-based assistance, find an attractive training partner, and 'attentively' spot their bench press."[66] That sounds provocative and fun and even as a driving force, yes?

Speaking of clever Australians, you may infer from a survey of Aussie individuals that libidinous *quantity* may have a *quality* all its own:

Consenting Australian adults in GenX have had an average of thirteen sexual partners in their lifetimes thus far (a mean average).[67] Aspiring Australian researchers, as women and *men at work*, seem to pursue interesting topics. Perhaps they should study the length of congressional sessions under the Southern Cross?

And there may be something to this thunder down under, according to the New Zealand Herald in a November 2016 article. A sex researcher named Andrea Pennington authored a book, *Orgasm Prescription For Women*, with the healthy assertion that ladies should enjoy three orgasms per week for their empowered self-esteem.

It is *aspirational* to think that steamy all-nighters happen all the time. Why did I assert the word *aspirational*? You may know that the motto for Harvard University, as the source of this performance fact, is *veritas* (truth).

- Five minutes is a statistical norm for the length of a congressional session.

Cinco minutos ... and that's the truth, as Lily Tomlin used to say on *Laugh In*.[68]

So, circle back to the idea of quality plus mutual pleasures in your state of the union. Don't worry *too much* about the length of your congressional session from foreplay to climax. Yet, bear in mind the statistical difference between average climax times for men and women...There truly *is* a difference of how men and women approach Sexercise:

- Males can quickly pursue and perform sexual intimacy to relax.
- Females need to relax (for longer) to perform intimately and climax.

Communication, empathy, and trust can lead to pleasure on both Mars and Venus. You may now know that one pleasure of mine is to learn where, when, and how certain words come to be. Here is how the words *sex*, *fornication*, and *f#&k* came about.

1. The original thirteenth-century meaning of *sex* simply meant genitalia. That makes me wonder about the saying, "I had sex." It's a bit of a wonder, as in, what happened to your junk, and where is it now?
2. *Fornication* stemmed from the ancient hangouts of prostitutes under arched entryways. *Fornix* literally means arch.
3. That four-letter word that starts with *f* and ends with *k* comes from an old German word, *ficken*, which meant to "strike or penetrate." That brings a new twist to a lucky strike, doesn't it? Now, let's have some sleepy "T."

NIGHTY NIGHT

Your lack of quality sleep can *lower* your production of free-form testosterone or "T" that stimulates muscle-building and libido in *both* sexes. Yup. Ladies need their testosterone production for some of the same biochemical reasons that men do, although normal testosterone production for ladies is about one-tenth of a gentleman's. "This (T) hormone also signals the body to make new blood cells, ensures that muscles and bones stay strong during and after puberty and enhances libido both in men and women."[69]

Think of testosterone (which is chemically the compound $C_{18}H_{28}O_2$) as your original and *natural* anabolic steroid. Can you guess what fat in our bodies helps generate it? If you guess cholesterol, you are correct. Cholesterol ain't all bad; Yet here comes a problem that is bad.

WHAT'S THE PROBLEM?

As Kelly Starrett pointedly told Tim Ferriss in *The Tools of Titans*, "If you wake up and you don't have a boner, there's a problem." That is a problem. A flagging flagstaff—the inability to rise to the occasion or a non-climactic finish line — can be symptomatic of cardiovascular disease in a guy. That's right, guys with erectile dysfunction (ED) have much *higher* risks of cardiac events.[70]

Guys, here is your climactic equation for health span and lifespan:

> Having sex twice a week means that a guy should live longer and better than one who passes muster only once a month.

Ladies, this isn't just an issue for Martian manhood. Don't views from Venus size up a dude's aesthetic body? Moving from eyes to aphrodisiacs, what's wrong with dark chocolate, oysters, and champagne? I also recommend garlic as a possible aphrodisiac if two are gonna tango.

FLYING SOLO

It doesn't *always* take two to tango. Woody Allen's screen character in *Annie Hall*, Alvy Singer, offered,

"Don't knock masturbation. It's sex with someone I love." Whether you fly united or not, sex can't be knocked when mind and body are aligned and engaged. Let's call your degree of mind-body-alignment an MBA in human factors.

GET IT ON WITH YOUR MBA.

Whether you like my suggestion of an MBA diploma or not, there *is* a credible linkage among GenX body image, sensuality, and sexuality.[71] Just as focused breathing and flow are tenets of yoga, proper positions are too. A downward dog *asana* (female) on the left of Figure 6.3 and a male's revolved triangle *asana* on the figure's right are MBA moves that can support mutually satisfying sexercise.

Many other *asanas* that promote satisfaction can be paired with classic partner positions. Think of a double boat pose or just use those flexible muscles and breaths in creative or steamy ways.

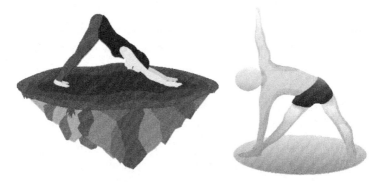

Figure 6.3: Get Your MBA. Downward Dog and Revolved Triangle Move for Sexercise

MISTER ED

Your generation may not remember a corny TV sitcom titled *Mr. Ed* from the 1960s (as I do). Yet, you should remember the valid findings for a prevalent "ED" finding for Mister GenX.

Guys, your physical activity, or PA, "has been identified as *the lifestyle factor most strongly correlated with erectile function* and the most important promoter of vascular health."[72] "Thus, moderate and vigorous-intensity PA is associated with *normal* erectile function and lower risk of ED."[73]

Ladies, I know in secondhand fashion and from firsthand research that your equal half of GenX has separate, significant sexual desires and sexual-drive challenges of your own.

Does that arouse your interest? One strong uplifter for modern times is that "Acute Exercise Improves Physical Sexual Arousal in Women Taking Antidepressants."[74] We know, quite sadly, how many women and men reported anxiety or depression before, during, and after COVID-19 struck. Their flows of dopamine, serotonin, and oxytocin beckoned for tune-ups. Even in the best of modern times, anxiety and depression affect too many Gen X health spans and lifespans.

Here's a tune-up candidate: work out to arouse pleasure and possibly take fewer prescription pills to dampen your angst. But wait, there is more than anxiety and depression dragging many GenX down:

"Obesity and inactivity have led to an increasing number of individuals with sexual dysfunctions (43 percent of women; 31 percent of men) ... Small bouts of exercise can drastically improve sexual functioning."[75]

So, get physical, both as a tribute to Olivia Newton-John and to your long and strong functional health spans, OK? Take two for your proofs positive.

CLIMACTIC RESULTS

A topic like sex is hard to skirt, as the Christian Bible, Madison Avenue (*Mad Men*) ads, Tik Tok™, and even classic writers mention it. Here are classic proof points:

- ✓ John Updike: "Sex is like money; only too much is enough."
- ✓ Woody Allen, as Alvy meeting with his therapist and wife, in *Annie Hall*:

  Therapist: "Do you have sex often?"
  Alvy: "Hardly ever…"
  Annie: "Constantly…"

I think that Alvy and Annie have a disconnect for expectations.

REALITY CHECK

"Go on doing what works for you and your honey. The take-home message … is that it's important to maintain a sexual *connection* with a romantic partner, but it is also important to have realistic expectations for one's sex life." [76]

SHAGGADELIC TRAINING

Here are select exercises, moves, and stretches to help a partner and you climb a magic mountain. If you don't enjoy mountain climbing, then linger and enjoy a Lotus on flat land. I repeat my kudos to Jason Rosell. He popularized certain exercises that can make pleasurable positions just so connected.

Think of your overall health span efforts in stamina, endured strength, and stretching or flexibility as worthy efforts for your sexercise. When you do sustain your complex moves, you are exercising for satisfying sex.

Here is just one heterosexual example. Yes, you probably read about the missionary position in a James Michener novel, *Hawaii*. As an aside, this old-fashioned *vanilla* position for congress may be one of the better couple positions for a female's vaginal climaxes.

But I digress ... Here are select exercises for GenX duos that just beckon with romping imagination and effort:

- Low, moderate, and high intensity "cardio" efforts
- Push-up Planks
- Buddy Back-to-back Sits
- Quadruped Planks
- Bench Presses (with or without a straddled spotter)
- Hip Thrusts
- Squats
- Down dog and donkey kicks.

There is *no* magic potion for sexercising. Just work together to improve your energetic capabilities for frolic.

Great gents do not reduce women and intimacy to sex alone. Sure, sex can and should be amazing. Yet, that shaggadelic act itself is a small numerator over the great denominators of your healthy intimate life. Girls, go along with Shania Twain, let it all hang out to have a good time. In that spirit, how about some non-trivial pursuits?

JUST SAYIN'

- A male's chance of death from sexual union is less than his chance of dying from a lightning strike.
- Good 'ol vibrators were invented in the 1880s for medical use *on males.*

- Modern males produce a lot less testosterone than did their ancestors.
- Modern women achieve climaxes about 60% of the time in heterosexual encounters.
- Sexual activity reduces migraine symptoms and boosts immunity.
- Only about one-fourth of congress is achieved with lights turned out.
- Four popes supposedly expired while engaged in flagrante delicto.
- Buzz Aldrin did *not* say "Good luck, Mr. Gorsky" on his historic moon walk in 1969. He debunked that fake news himself, although one could sense how this comment might have inspired him to achieve greatness. This is the origin and context: Aldrin's childhood neighbor, Mrs. Gorsky, told her husband: "*You'll get oral sex when that kid next door walks on the moon.*"

EUREKA! THE BENCH PRESS

You've now come across this chapter's focus strength move: the bench press, that I just mentioned in a list of great strength moves for sexercise. Some resistance moves can sound a bit mysterious, like the Zottman curl, for example. Others can be suggestive, like a skull crusher. The bench press is a straightforward, or rather, a supine-upward exercise term.

Your supine position for a bench press means that your nose and knees are pointed to the ceiling or sky from your position on a weight bench. This is the *opposite orientation* to your prone position. A *press* is a push-upward motion. Look for a sturdy and safe bench, *with or without a straddle spotter*, and find a rack mechanism to stow your loaded barbell if you are using a barbell for your bench presses. (Yes, like many other strength exercises, you can substitute two dumbbells for the single barbell in the bench press.) If you are not using a barbell, then you have no worries about the rack. Remember, safety first—with or without a spotter or coach. *No Bench?* Adapt.

If you *don't* have a weight bench handy, you can *floor press* with dumbbells without too much compromise in your up-pressing workload. You get the upper half of your pushing motion and can make the downward eccentric phase of each floor press good enough.

Bench presses are held in high regard by power-lifting organizations. Although the bench press is *not* an Olympic lift, it is one of the three competitive powerlifts, complementing the deadlift and the back squat for the recognized *power three.*

Here are safety and performance points for your bench press technique:

1. Lie flat on your back on a bench.
2. Grip the bar with your hands just wider than shoulder-width apart, so when you're at the bottom of your move, your hands are directly above your elbows. This allows for maximum force generation.
3. Bring the bar slowly down to your chest as you breathe in.
4. Gripping the barbell hard, push up as you breathe out. Watch a spot on the ceiling rather than the bar, so you can ensure it travels the same path every time.

PRESS POINTS

- Your feet should stay on the ground beneath or behind your knees. Press your feet into the floor to create tension in your core, hamstrings, and glutes.
- Your head, shoulders, and hips should all remain on the bench throughout the lift.
- Your shoulders should retract and press firmly into the bench to create a solid foundation.

THE SETUP

- Your eyes should be directly under the barbell, and the bar should be no higher than your wrists when your arms are locked out overhead.
- For most people, your hands should be on the bar just a bit wider apart than your shoulders. Yes, there are grip-width variations with which to progress, as I S.A.I.D.

UNRACK AND RERACK

- Use a spotter! If you don't have one, stop well before failure so that you can safely rerack the bar.
- To *un*rack the bar, start with a strong lock-out where the bar is directly above your shoulders.
- Lower the bar under control for one or two seconds to approximately where a chest strap heart-rate monitor would be, then press until your elbows are straight and you have the bar under control.
- Rerack carefully and make sure the bar is secure before you release the tension in your arms.

Yes, you can vary the angle of many weight benches. I prefer to use an angled bench for dumbbell shoulder presses, but I stay with a flat bench for my power bench presses.

Each bench press repetition and set challenge your chest, back, shoulders, and arms to elevate heavy weights. You can check online with the International Powerlifting Federation or similar powerlifting organizations to gauge what champions who "approach the bench" can do.

Please approach the bench and push it, "push it real good." As a takeaway, please judge this: Prepping for and enjoying Kamasutra motions is good GenXercise. Bench pressing is such prepping. If it feels good, do it. You just might rise to the top of the charts!

Or, as Salt-N-Pepa sang in 1986, "Show the guys that we know how to become number one in a hot party show." That is one kind of result. Now, turn the page to read about the results of your strength work. It is always good to keep the end result and goal of your lifts, pushes, pulls, twists, and carries in your sight. TINA.

Results ...
Period.

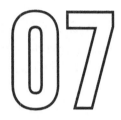

If my forebear, Emerson, was alive today, I do not doubt that he would
have written of believing "men *and* women." Of that inclusion, I am
certain. Be strong, ladies and gentlemen. Be a great believer in root
causes and ultimate effects.

Let's get serious here, very serious about your end results. Those
lasting results from your regular, focused, and timed resistance efforts.
You have read my singular emphases ending with a Period or TINA
in prior pages. As in, move heavy stuff, *die harder.* Period.

As a systems engineer in my prior life, I knew about transformation.
And I learned how to process that makeover for the systems my teams
engineered. Think about the results of exercise-induced sweat and
systematic inflammation as a system. If you think that inflammation
is totally a negative factor in systems, think again. As in Figure 7.1,
think cause and effect.

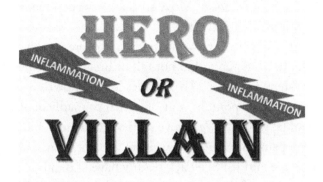

Figure 7.1: Inflammation Causes What?

NECESSARY TEARS

As I wrote for a 2022 *NFPT* article, "inflammation supports either balanced, normal activity, or in excess, triggers a tipping point for abnormal physical (and medical) conditions. The benefit of 'collateral damage' from microtears generated by training efforts to improve strength is an example of when the inflammatory process serves a necessary purpose."

It is your GenX mission to benefit from that inflammatory collateral damage. Your gains are triggered by muscle *microtears*.

CAUSE AND EFFECT

The cause: Certain muscular actions cause bodily inflammation.

The repair process: Your skeletal muscles naturally restore, rebuild, and revitalize or grow (with the assistance of proper diet and appropriate rest, of course).

The lasting effect: You will achieve a healthy physical return on your investment of regular lifting, pushing, pulling, and carrying things. Think of longer and thicker sarcomeres. Think of sturdier skeletal bones. And imagine scores of health span and lifespan reasons.

Why loiter, linger, or languish? Move stuff as very good medicine—stat. Greater yet, move *heavy* stuff.

Get your strong-to-save work underway before you give away your muscle fiber to sarcopenia. Do not fall or break a bone because your muscular system and poor MBA grades let you down.

Do *not* get to the point in your life when you sadly realize that you woulda, coulda, yet you *didn't* move stuff as good medicine. Don't wait to clear menopause or *manopause* waivers. Do not delay with "yes, but" reasons that Joe and Jill Six-Pack readily have at hand.

Their "yes, buts" do not please me, and those excuses do not put them in good standing with Jedis. Rather, be a Jedi knight or a Princess Leia who ascribes to this challenge: "Do or do not. There is no try."

Strength or resistance training results are your physical banking cornerstone. Results that help you down age to die harder and later. Do it now yet do it deliberately.

NOT SO FAST

Slower lifting *can* be better, with metabolic strength exercises to maximize or *max out* the times under tension (TuT) that your muscles endure. You read earlier about a one-minute pull-up as a bad-ass benchmark of endured strength. Now, think about lifting, pushing, pulling, twisting, or carrying a fairly heavy object for at least ninety seconds without pauses at isometric points in your repetitive motions in slow sets.

Ninety to 120 seconds of slow repetitions per set is a type of metabolic resistance lifting. Think of a seven to eight second half of your goblet squat in the downward eccentric phase. Then, without a pause at the isometric bottom of this exercise, slowly rise to the up position in seven to eight seconds as you exhale. Repeat about five times until the ninety seconds have elapsed. That is a metabolic conditioning routine to remember.

A key point: only minimal rest is allowed between your metabolic exercise sets of resistance moves. With appropriate weights as resistance, you feel a good burn as you increase insulin sensitivity and promote your muscle-building hormonal signals. As a student of your D.E.E.P. endeavor, you can choose this occasional *King TuT* variant of strength training for your bespoke training goal. Your trainer, workout buddy, or you in solo formation will choose among many workout protocols with different timing guidelines.

As Andy Galpin, PhD, advises on his Train Heroic website, the choice of slow reps versus fast reps in a set *depends* on your specific outcomes. Each protocol has a special purpose that starts with you and your intended results.

Example. You may choose a forty- to seventy-second set time for a muscle hypertrophy workout to grow your muscle size in an eight-to-twelve-week periodization. The focused amount of time spent on each set will be dictated by the resistance load and your strength level.

To reinforce these result-oriented words in your fitness primer, consider Figure 7.2 below.

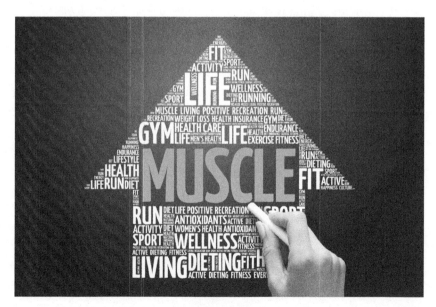

Figure 7.2: Draw Your Results, Journal
Them, Then Move Stuff

PLAN YOUR EXECUTION, EXECUTE YOUR PLAN

Reminder: when your strength movements or exercises begin to feel easy, it's time to raise the stakes. Do keep this two-by-two guideline in mind as you progress through your strength periodization. You can increase the resistance/weight for a certain exercise once you can perform two more repetitions beyond your repetition goal for the last set for two weeks in a row. This isn't Noah's Ark, yet it a fine 2 by 2 milestone.

So, challenge your muscles and mind to tackle more volume or intensity, or shift the tempo of your movement. When you do, favorable results follow. Period.

For example: You are in a hypertrophy and strength mesocycle. You note that you can lift a previously "heavy" load twelve times in your sets when you planned for ten repetitions per set. At the H & S limit of twelve repetitions, you are ready to increase your resistance by 5 to 10 percent for a next overload cycle. Does that sound like a workable two by two plan? It should.

It is not an epiphany when I state this: *Hope is not a valid plan or second-half strategy for you.*

To get the most out of your strength and complementary stamina training, you must do the work for health span and lifespan. Do you remember those volume, intensity, and tempo factors for strength workouts from earlier pages of Strong to Save? Let's add one more factor for another 4-letter word. That fourth word is Adapt or Adjust. Why? Because ship happens in my Navy parlance, or stuff happens per Murphy's Laws of fitness. So, V,I,T becomes **VITA** for your life. **Adapt** to new exercises and adjust them to keep the workout session fresh and exciting.[77]

Let's augment this *A* of your dolce VITA.

ADAPT AND ADOPT

Remember Bill Bowerman's assertion about athletes? Nearly everyone can and should pursue the health benefits of strength training. Some who suffer from limited movement, either because of age or because of physical injury, may decide it is hard or impossible to exercise efficiently. Folks do not let something hard or seemingly impossible stand in your way. Adapt to become the very best that you can be. How about adoption?

If you are looking to adopt a checklist of great GenX strength results, look no further than this table. *Unless otherwise indicated, a benchmark is the same for both genders.*

1. Hold a single leg stand position with your eyes closed for twenty seconds. Be sure to do this unilaterally on either leg at a time to prove your spatial awareness is *not* one-sided.
2. Grip a dynamometer to impulsively generate a strong pressure reading in ~ 3 to 5 seconds (with different levels for gender and age).
   • Work on your hand and arm strength to be strong as someone ten years younger than you in calendar years. That difference in *fitness years* is great for both genders.
3. Perform a sit-to-rise test without using your hands.
4. Do Turkish get-ups with a heavy weight or kettlebell.
5. Walk with a heavy weight in each hand for thirty paces as a farmer does.
6. Complete a single pull-up in ~30-60 seconds.
   • Note that women are now encouraged to pursue pull-ups that were once considered to be the sole province of men.
7. Row a 500-meter distance on an indoor rower, with a finish time in the top 10 percent of your decade age group.
8. Hold a bear crawl plank position for ninety seconds.
9. Hold a forearm plank position for three minutes.

10. Guys—do twenty push-ups with good form; ladies—do ten push-ups with good form.
11. Optimize your natural, nasal breathing to liberate "Doctor NO" (nitric oxide) for endured strength achievements.
12. Expand your lung capacity and use your pneumatic pumping system to exhale rapidly.

Yes, down-aging criteria numbers eleven and twelve might be considered more as bedrock stamina criteria for your physical bank than cornerstone strength. Yet, I know of *no* great GenX for strength who exhibits *subpar* lung capacity. *And there was that 12–13-minute finish line that you considered in the Sexercise chapter.*

For extra credit as a number thirteen, you can break your dark chocolate bar into four pieces and eat only one, as Judith Viorst challenged. Are you ready for your next lost and found?

EUREKA! BATTLE ROPE FUNCTIONAL TRAINING

You've reached this chapter's focused strength effort: battle rope functional training.

The heavier the rope's weight and the longer its length, the more intensity you will experience. The double slap technique (shown in Figure 7.3) is your best motion for intervals or high-intensity training results with your new friend – the battle rope. Try other slap techniques – like alternating sides – to mix up this valuable functional training.

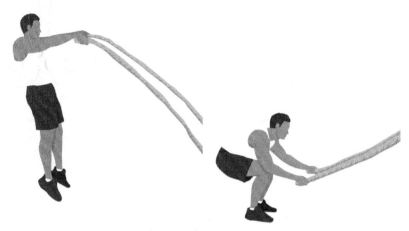

Figure 7.3: Battle Rope for Strength and Stamina

Kudos to you, my great GenX practitioner. You've now consumed the first seven chapters of your GenX fit map.

But wait, there are more X factors to help you move stuff in your way for another forty to fifty years. Please note that I limited chapter 8's X factors to things that I know well or have experienced. There are certainly more dietary, ergogenic, integrative medicines, and training aids "out there."

Remember that I implore you to be a student of your endeavors. I implore you to build your own physical banking portfolio with out-of-the-ordinary factors that help you stay strong to save.

Before you turn the page, highlight these closing remarks by Mark Rippetoe and Socrates about weak people and amateurs:

"Strong people are harder to kill than weak people and are more useful in general" (Mark Rippetoe).

"No one has a right to be an amateur in the matter of physical training" (Socrates).

Be far more useful and avoid being an amateur your great GenX factors.

Yes, you can and should!

Your X Factors

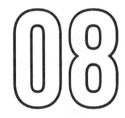

"Nearly everyone dies before they're ready."

—Tim Ferriss, author, Tools of Titans

D o not be "everyone." Be *the one* who defies odds.

A great GenX certainly works to avert an early arrival at heaven's gate. 'Tis far better to *reach* your final resting place after an added decade of vital health span. Yes, you can! You can with strength work, good and learned practices, and with a little bit of luck.

Thank goodness for natural boosters and enablers for your extended second-half performance. Yes, enablers from nature and technology abound to help you defy and defer the pearly gates. *Die harder and cheat death for longer* and have more fun during your earthly journey.

Do your strength training consistently as if your life depended on it. That is because *it does.*

1. Surround yourself with folks and resources to fortify your physical bank and make your savings persist.
2. Become a practical student of what it takes to win at the game of a longer and better life. Do bear in mind what Derek Sivers offered in *Tools of Titans*: "It's not what you know, it is *what you do consistently.*"

Take consistent habitual action to maintain your skeletal muscle mass as a matter of added life and mojo.

This chapter cites provocative and useful boosters from both old-fashioned nature and newfangled technology that help you on your strength journey. Once again, moving heavy stuff is great medicine for your second-half performance and a fine investment in your physical bank. So, let's consider tangible tune-ups to help you move it, move it. Ready, set, go with the twenty-fourth letter of our English alphabet, and currently the favorite letter of one Elon Musk…

X

You may recall Simon Cowell's *X Factor* entertainment show. That *X Factor* title implied *in*tangible "things" that enabled *star* quality.

Your own X factors are also strong stuff, yet they are *tangible* rather than intangible differentiators. So, boost your *starring* strength with extraordinary enablers.

You now know that resistance or strength moves, done *consistently*, are medicinal factors to die harder. Your functional strengths make you an *Xercist* who:

- ✓ banishes chronic stress,
- ✓ limits white fat accumulation,
- ✓ improves insulin sensitivity,
- ✓ boosts key anti-inflammatory glutathione,
- ✓ reduces testosterone-limiting factors,
- ✓ promotes Sexercise moves in superior ways,
- ✓ boosts your immunities to offset or counter external and internal stressors that life presents.

Are you ready to study and apply these recommended strength boosters as a card-carrying Xercist?

X-RATED BOOSTER CLUB

Eight subchapters follow with one X Factor each as a titan's tool for you. These 8 segments flesh out your fit map with natural and technology *strength boosters*.

Notes: One prospective strength factor, synthetic anabolic steroids, is my *off-limits* no-no. Remember the Netflix documentary, *Icarus*, and the exposed Russian doping scandals? This show is worth watching to grasp why 'roids are not the way to become strong to save. Another performance enhancer that isn't worth your risks, in my opinion, is amphetamines. No-no.

There is *no* primacy for the order of these X Factor subchapters. Some are inherently longer than others, yet all are intended to help you boost your performance. None are encyclopedic, exhaustive dealings. It is up to you to smartly search, select, and savor your own X factors. Here are those eight enablers that work for me and are summarized for you:

1. Natural ergogenic supplements.
2. Timing factors and chronotypes.
3. Mimicking Morpheus with regular restorative sleep.
4. Making mobility matter—with supportive stability and stretching to maintain your "original" strengths.
5. Health devices and appliances—both analog and digital.
6. Breath and breathing.
7. Natural integrative medicines (IM).
8. Xformers.

Themes of this overall chapter and its segments are shown where *X* marks the spot in Figure 8.1.

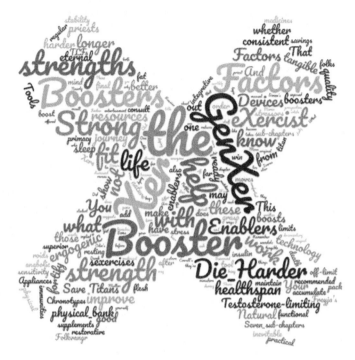

Figure 8.1 Your Strong to Save X Factors

You won the coin toss, so be ready to receive in your strong second half, naturally.

SUBCHAPTER 1—NATURAL ERGOGENICS

Let's start with good-ol' nutrients from mother earth. That is, after I share what the meaning of a natural (legal) ergogenic is.

An ergo(work) genic(promoter) can be a tool, a food, a food supplement, or some other enabler that helps you perform better. Think of caffeine or an electrolyte drink, a "safe" creatine supplement, or a protein drink as safe and legal ergogenics. You can and should also think of mental boosters like meditation and focused breathing as ergogenic aids.

Natural ergogenics help you down age.

Organic macronutrients and micronutrients, plus clean water fuel, are what boost your strong motions as medicine. What could stand in your way? Many things can. Consider these five barriers that challenge your strong, natural fueling efforts: 1.) poor topsoil, 2.) convenience foods, 3.) age-related absorption, 4.) micronutrient imbalances, and 5.) key vitamin deficiencies.

1. Our topsoil *isn't* what it used to be. Sadly, Vitamin P(lant) gets to your plate and palate with lesser quantity and quality than prior generations enjoyed in their crops and produce. *I use Vitamin P to depict plant-based, essential micronutrients to stay strong to save.*

    As you and I age, our absorption of essential "micros" *lessens,* whatever is the quantity or quality on your plate. So, be very, very attentive as you advance your health span. *Act* to optimally absorb your Vitamin P and key minerals whatever your calendar age.

2. Complacency can set in for empty nesters and middle-aged folks. Convenience food, that is too accessible in my book, is rarely as nutritious as your carefully planned home-cooked meals. And by carefully, I mean that you should limit processed foodstuffs when dining out *or* eating in! If a human made it, *don't* eat it ... as Jack LaLanne advised.

3. Generation X *should* live longer than my generation (that is, *if* we can control obesity, viruses, and opioid epidemics). Aging brings poorer food absorption along with it, even when you are a great GenX. So, your bodily absorption of nutrients will *drop* for many years as calendar years mount. Remember, it is your goal to extend your health span, so commit to fueling your body for that extra decade or so of both health span and lifespan. Make each month a micronutrient month to journal

and celebrate. If you do not, marginal "micro" deficiencies may also extend with unsavory and unhealthy results.

4. Imbalances. You probably ingest *more* sodium and calcium than your grandparents did. You likely consume *less* vitamin C, potassium, and magnesium than they did. And so, you need to balance your physical banking accounts with nutrients like they did—if you intend to down age.

5. A lack of key micronutrients. "Deficiencies in … iron, iodine, Vitamin A, folate, and Zinc can have *devastating consequences*."[78]

    What's a strong GenX to do to avoid *devastating consequences?* You will need to have far better answers than "I really don't know" or "that's life."

Please stay with me as to find truth and to shun those devastating consequences. Get ready to produce.

If you are not Grecian or a language expert, the X factor *ergonomic* comes from the two terms *ergon* (work) and *gennan* (to produce).

- Vitamins and minerals, as vital micronutrients, are practical work producers and boosters of health for all of us.

Yes, you should consider key supplementation if you are a vegan, if you have diabetes, and *when* you are an *athlete.* Training and eating are necessarily different for great, athletic folks like you. Remember that a natural byproduct of your exercise to sweat is oxidative free radicals or ROS. Vitamin P is a prime-time *counter* to ROS. Trust dietary experts and count on me.

Let's start with a baker's dozen (13) of vitamins and minerals to counter-attack inflammation, stress, and ROS. Did you know that a Polish researcher named Funk coined the term vita(life) min(amine)? He (wrongly) thought that amino acids composed our tiny life-supporting substances, our vitamins. Such is life.

Now, consider the *Dietary Guidelines for Americans*, eighth edition (2015–2020)[79] which offers you three solid nutritional tips:

- Focus on your *needed* nutrients as a uniquely strong athlete, including "right" absorbed amounts of potassium, calcium, vitamin D, vitamin B12, minerals, and dietary fiber.
- Lose weight or maintain a healthy weight.
- Meet individual calorie and nutrition needs to help maintain energy levels.

A great Gen X takes these 3 tips – nutrition needs, lean body composition, and energy levels – for that MBA degree.

If *Strong to Save* was an unabridged work instead of a lean primer or fit map, you'd certainly read more flex alerts about the merits of clean, anti-inflammatory eating to boost your strength and vitality. Take one.

Here is just one example of a much-needed micronutrient mineral. The mineral *zinc* must be absorbed at sufficient levels that vary by gender and age, or else. Whatever your GenX age or sex, you forego proper zinc absorption at your own peril.

Reasons for proper zinc absorption include:

- Full function of the immune system, including eyesight, as zinc helps filter high energy blue and UV rays from our sun
- Correct DNA synthesis and cell division
- Protect your cells from oxidative damage that is stress induced from life, smoking, excess sun or exercise (RoS)
- Properly metabolize fatty acids
- Metabolize macronutrient proteins, carbohydrates, and fats.

✓ Zinc is called a *micro*nutrient for good reason, as a "healthy" adult American has *only* about 2 grams of zinc stored in skeletal muscles and bones.[80] Oh, what a difference 2 absorbed grams make!

For emphases, maintain those 2 grams of zinc to:

✓ counter exercise-induced oxidative damage (ROS),
✓ lower adult Diabetes in rural areas (yes, zip codes unfortunately matter),
✓ inhibit age-related macular degeneration (AMD),
✓ assist in protein synthesis, and
✓ aid your virility functions too. Oysters are considered aphrodisiacs due in part to their high zinc concentration. In fact, oysters are the most concentrated food source of zestful zinc.

Notes: As zinc *isn't* concentrated in fruits and vegetables, lifestyle vegetarians may well need zinc supplements.

As you will read for other minerals and supplements, there are timing issues to ingest zinc for your best bodily absorption. It is wise to separate your ingestion of zinc foods or supplements ingestion of magnesium or soaking in Epsom salt baths, as your equally vital magnesium (Mg) absorption may be adversely impacted.[81]

MG SPEAK

As a great safeguard, your dietary supplementation will likely include magnesium too, as it is vital to countless bodily functions. *Highlight this:* Too many, perhaps 70 percent or more of GenX, are deficient in bodily absorption for this key mineral.

I flag another chemical advisory for your MBA here: scientists tell us that there are seven types of magnesium compounds that a healthy person absorbs to support nerves, muscles, and sleep. Ingest and absorb *all* of those 7 magnesium compounds from natural Vitamin P and/or from supplements. Mg notes:

A. Magnesium levels should be checked in your annual blood tests. Don't skip a chance to monitor your biochemistry in action, please. Just remember that there can be a difference between serum levels from that annual test and absorbed cellular levels of key nutrients, including Mg.

B. Some people may have gut issues from Magnesium supplements. One MG compound, magnesium citrate, helps gut absorption and healthy bacteria colonies grow. So, it is imperative to know how your gut and you get along with Magnesium from food and supplements.

"MICRO" BANKING

I reemphasize that you are unique, so your own physical micro banking is also unique. Table 8.1 *generically* summarizes key vitamins and minerals as your candidates for healthy micronutrition from food and supplements. Your needs may differ, so stay vigilant as a student of your nutritional endeavors and adapt, as necessary, to live long and prosper.

FLEX ALERT #24:

Try nature first and trusted supplementation second.

I am *not* a fan of multivitamins for athletes, with the exception of AREDS2* eye vitamins to protect against macular degeneration and vision loss as you advance in calendar years.

I *am* a proponent of discrete and trusted supplements when and if a regular blood lab test shows a debit in that account of your physical bank. Or, when you exhibit common symptoms from one or more nutrient deficiency(ies). As we just highlighted zinc as one vital nutrient, consider these common symptoms of Zn deficiency:

1. hair loss.
2. changes in smoothness of coloration of finger and toenails.
3. diarrhea.
4. prone to more inflammation or bodily infections.
5. feeling irritable.
6. loss of appetite.
7. impotence.
8. eye problems.

No doubt you can see why zinc is darned important for health span and lifespan.

*Notes AREDS is the acronym for Age-Related Eye Disease Study. AREDS 2 supplements, which I take regularly when I break my fast, contain vital vitamins and minerals to promote your eye function and vision.

Our National Eye Institute reminds you and me to:

> "talk with your doctor before you start taking a new medicine or supplement — and tell them about all the other medicines, vitamins, and supplements you take."

My GP and optometrist want me to supplement with AREDS2. Some folks may experience slight gut issues, due to the potency of some AREDS2 ingredients. As always, trust, yet verify your unique response to food and supplements. Timing is one unique response.

TIME PASSAGES

It may take weeks to get your body boosted to "healthy" levels of *some* micronutrients if you are found to be deficient. Good things take time. And good things for you come in small, timely packages.

Conversely, it can take weeks for your body to "detoxify" too much of good things absorbed – like iron. Study this micronutrient overview as you remember that great timing is about as important as quantity.

PEEKING AT MICRONUTRIENTS

Micronutrient	Detailed Peek
Vitamin C	250 milligrams (mg)/day *The government's <u>recommended daily allowance</u> for older women is 75 mg, and 90 mg for men.*
Vitamin D3	1000 IU / day Fifteen to twenty minutes of solar exposure daily is a *natural* way to generate some of this vital micronutrient. *If immunity is a pressing issue, as is the case for rhinovirus and novel coronavirus (COVID), this 1000 IU level might be raised. Check what Dr. Anthony Fauci takes daily.*
Vitamin E	A normal diet *may* suffice for adequate absorption of this fat-soluble vitamin.
Note for Vitamin B-12	*If an elder is a vegetarian or not eating proper, energy-dense macronutrients; vitamin B-12 could be deficient too.*
Calcium (Ca)	Take 400 mg/day (Older clients generally gain adequate calcium from dairy and other macro-nutrient sources). *Some* older women have an extraordinary need for calcium absorption to maintain bone density after menopause. Calcium and vitamin D3 are complementary micronutrients for optimal absorption.
Iron (Fe)	*Normal* Macronutrient diets are adequate for older clients' iron (Fe) levels. *The <u>livingto100 calculator</u> credibly advises that excess retained iron is a detriment to long life, particularly for males.*
Magnesium (Mg)	**400 milligrams(mg)/day** *Most* older clients *fail to absorb adequate* magnesium. *Note: Blood draws may not accurately measure cellular absorption of this vital mineral.*

Micronutrient	Detailed Peek
Selenium (SE)	55 micrograms (μ/day) This *tiny* level should not be underestimated. Its metabolic role is key for a master's athletic performances.
Sodium (Na)	Note this salty exception is to *reduce* ingestion for *most* clients! Most older clients ingest *more* than their MDRs of 2.3 grams of salt per day. Concerns of hypertension and metabolic syndrome (MetS) are high when excess sodium is retained.
L-Carnitine	**Take** 2–6 grams per day (if needed). Vegetarians' Doctors may find a want or need for this amino acid supplementation.
Ubiquinol—CoQ10	Take 200 mg/day. As our bodily generation of this heart-healthy micronutrient drops notably with age, a professional might suggest supplementation.
Zinc (Zn)	Take 11 mg/day. Zinc is essential for good vision, libido, and immunity.
Other Considerations	One reason why it takes years to become a registered dietitian is the practical knowledge for undesirable side-effects—such as for calcium and vitamin D interactions. Whole food ingestion is usually superior to ergogenics or supplements as a first order for getting those micronutrients "banked." It is good to remember that four key vitamins for clients of all ages (A, D, E, and K) need fatty acids ("healthy fat") for optimal absorption. Blood-test lab results may not reflect true cellular absorption. Professional advice should be considered.

Table 8.1 Peeking at your Vital Micronutrients

Are you set to consider the strong impact of your great GenX internal factors?

YOUR ATHLETE WITHIN

Experienced and elite athletes, perhaps including the current you, assuredly watch their diets. And most top-end athletes *do* take supplements in their pursuits of peak performance.[82]

If endured strength is your game, consider what supplement a Tour de France's team physician insisted that his riders take. His endurance riders consume an upper level (UL) of vitamin D. Right, that sunshine micronutrient is prescribed to counter inflammation or immune-system compromises for their muscles, cardio-respiratory systems, and brains.

Like those endurance athletes, we appreciate just enough or "friendly" muscular system inflammation for gains. However, we don't need the "foe" or villain levels that a highly trained GenX can face.[83]

Nutri-fact scientists offer this attention grabber:

"Marginal deficiency may *only* be apparent
when the metabolic rate is high."[84]

Isn't it a paradox that your great, healthy, sweaty activities can have a "flip side" of unhealthy potential? You know that I *want you* to get your metabolic rate high. Yet, I don't want you to overtrain to produce villainous levels of inflammation and cytokine flows. Certainly, you *don't* want to overtrain to identify marginal deficiencies in nutrients. Thank goodness for natural boosters and enablers to offset those high effects of your sweat and toil.

As a great GenX who is accustomed to high exertion, you will face marginal nutrient deficiencies at some point or points in your strength journey. I implore you to get your metabolism clicking at a high level. When you do, you may find performance benefits from safe ergogenics (meaning in solid and liquid form.) "Doctor, Doctor, Mister M.D." is one of those resources that a great GenX will recruit and retain.

Please tell your doctor about any supplements and medications that you are taking – both prescribed and over-the-counter substances. Here is a Q and A to underscore why?

> Q: Why did the actor in the prescription drug commercial cross the road?
> A: To get to the other side effects.

Potential side effects or interactions with medications you may take can and do happen. Medications are certainly available and seem to be readily prescribed these days. *Do you absolutely need any or all those "meds"?* That is my rhetorical question to help avoid "some" polypharmacy that is costly and unnatural. And, as you will soon read in another X Factor segment, there are many natural products that may suffice.

Here is an important, cautionary note: The US Food and Drug Administration (FDA) treats supplements quite differently than it does for food and drug regulations. Therefore,

- each supplement manufacturer is responsible for the safety and proper labeling of its products. You may trust, yet you *must* verify the quality of any supplements that you take. *Never* buy or take supplements that are not "third party" tested and analyzed for quality and purity. 'Tis sad yet true, once again, that P.T. Barnum was right about suckers. Don't be a sucker.

Else, you may play truth or consequences with high stakes.

I am a proponent of "some" ergogenics and supplements. Perhaps you are or will become a proponent too. Caffeine is one ergogenic that we will soon consider. *When* I drink caffeine, and how it affects my performance is a timing factor I keep conscious. I am confident that caffeine improves my mind-muscle performance. Yet I know that caffeine may affect my gut and bladder on occasion. Be mindful of the adverb "may" in your next Flex Alert.

FLEX ALERT #25:

"The timing of caffeine, nitrates, and creatine monohydrate *may* impact outcomes such as exercise performance, strength gains and other exercise training adaptations."[85] Trust, perhaps, yet verify—always.

NATURAL SUPPLEMENTS AND STIMULANTS

Sports nutritionists regularly address natural ergogenics *vis a vis* their quantity, timing, and potential performance benefits. This list is *not* all-inclusive. Yet these cited "athletic" supplements will give you a foundational knowledge of foods, essential oils, and even lifestyle habits that produce results for you. Are you ready for a naturally healthy jolt from caffeine?

COFFEE

Best-selling author Michael Pollan evaluated a once-obscure African shrub that helped to turn night into day for the Industrial Revolution. You might consider adding *Caffeine: How Coffee and Tea Created the Modern World* to your self-gifted book or audiobook list.

That shrub's berries, when processed, are a natural stimulant with situational health benefits. Some researchers suggest that coffee drinkers are more active than non-java drinkers.[86]

The caffeine in coffee (or tea) blocks the receptors of your neurotransmitter, *adenosine*, while increasing *dopamine* and other happy hormones in your brain. Also, antioxidants in coffee—called *polyphenol* and *flavonoids*—increase your insulin sensitivities, counter inflammation, and noticeably boost your metabolism. When drunk in moderation (as in *only* three 6-ounce cups daily) coffee may *lower* your risks of strokes, dementia-related diseases, depression, and cognitive declines.

After moderation and timing, here is another coffee-and-tea caveat:

caffeine has a long *half-life* in your body.

Daytime caffeine may still be stimulating you at night. That banked stimulus may lower your amount of rapid eye movement (REM) sleep, keep your heart rate elevated, and lower your heart rate variability when you are trying to achieve restorative sleep for your mind and body. Recall that *higher* heart rate variabilities (HRV) are good as your feed and restore systems counter cortisol and stressful fight or flight factors.

And did you know that blonde- or medium-roast coffees may have higher caffeine concentrations than do bold or robust coffees? Check for yourself. Could you live with a diluted cuppa or drink decaffeinated coffee if you must have some after your dinner? As an important side note—alcohol in a coffee drink, even a small aperitif, also has a metabolic half-life that can awaken you, elevate your temperature, lower your HRV, and raise your heart rate in the wee hours to adversely impact your sleep.

TEA

As the natural stimulant (caffeine) is common with coffee, some of tea's health benefits were just highlighted. One added benefit of some trusted source teas is one special *polyphenol*, or *tea catechin*, called EGCG that counters those reactive oxygen species (ROS) that are byproducts of smoking, pollution, sun damage, and exercise. Know how to counter ROS as a byproduct of moderate to intense exercises (like weightlifting).

Think of ROS as an "exercise rust" that must be countered with antioxidants like EGCG if you are to restore your body for a next workout session. *Moi?* I do drink tea. When in Ireland, I drink what the thirsty Irish drink the most (which *isn't* Guinness by the way.)

Tannic acids in some tea brands can bother my empty stomach. As an occasional alternative, I take trusted-source green tea pills to boost my catechins to fight inflammation and counter postexercise ROS.

- As a buyer-beware caution, you may see EGCG on a tea supplement bottle listed as a "fat burner." You would need to consume a whole lot of green tea pills to lose appreciable pounds. Caveat Emptor!

SODAS/ENERGY DRINKS

I am a *nonfan* of sodas and most energy drinks. Their sugar or artificial sweetener contents, stimulant levels, and additives are not attractive to me, even if they might improve my athletic performances.

I want to be there at the finish line of my journey by hydrating naturally and skipping unnatural stimulants. I drink sparkling water with a twist of lemon or lime as my alternative to sodas and energy drinks. Or, as you've already read, I drink coffee or tea moderately.

CREATINE MONOHYDRATE

A counseling point from the respected Mayo Clinic:

> creatine *might* benefit athletes who need short
> bursts of speed or increased muscle strength, such as
> sprinters, weightlifters, and team sport athletes.

Why? Creatine is a natural amino acid that is found mostly in your body's muscles and brain. Your liver, pancreas, and kidneys can make about 1 gram of creatine per day in prime times. One gram – or a *quarter* teaspoon. That production becomes *inadequate* in middle age to help offset sarcopenia for many folks.

Please acknowledge facts of creeping biochemical inefficiencies as time passes in your life-- even as a great GenX. Our internal factories just do not produce enough key substances – like testosterone, creatine, or Coenzyme Q10 – as examples.

Taking creatine monohydrate orally might *or* might not help you, yet evidence suggests that it won't hinder your health span or lifespan *if it is taken as directed*. When used orally at appropriate doses, creatine is likely to be *safe* for up to about five years of ingestion. It is important to choose a creatine product that follows recommended manufacturing practices and subscribes to third-party testing to (hopefully) ensure its high quality.

A possible side effect of this creatine supplement is weight gain for added muscle size and retained water weight. Remember the likelihood of side effects and the half-life of safe supplemental gain. Let's shift to healthy acids, *not* psychedelic ones.

"GOOD" FATTY ACIDS

Try to consume "good" fats and fatty acids at the rate of about half a gram of fat per pound of body weight. This guideline is true for *both* ladies and gentlemen. In my terms, good fats are ergogenic.

What is a healthy fat? Healthy fats are technically called monounsaturated or polyunsaturated fats on your food labels. Think of avocados, wild salmon, and nuts as natural sources of these healthy fats. These foods offer a good Omega-3 to Omega-6 ratio of 1:4 or lower. Conversely, "bad" fats are technically labeled as *trans* fats or *saturated* fats. Those evil fats can be found in chicken skin, fatty "marbled" red meats, whole-fat dairy products, and lard. Beware of a food label that hides "zombie" fats in its total fat contents.

If the food label is on a human-made or processed food item, it may hide an unhealthy zombie fat. Think of these hidden, unhealthy fats in terms of higher LDL levels and lower levels of "good" HDLs in your cardiovascular system. Remember, America's number-one killer is CVD and atherosclerosis. Further, remember that one respected medical doctor asserted that **the normal American diet was our number one cause of morbidity.** Oy!

Here is your quick homework assignment to avoid the zombie-fat connection with morbidity, in the spirit of Jack LaLanne and trusted medical science. Choose a processed food product's label with which to play Sherlock Holmes. Look at the total fat entry on the label. Then, add up all the healthy and unhealthy types of fat that are listed on the label. If the sum of the sub listings is less than the total fat of a product, then unhealthy hidden or zombie fats are probably present yet *un*accounted for.

Zombie fats include partially hydrogenated shortening or partially hydrogenated fat and oils. These unnatural oils are doubly vexing for your heart. Zombie fats raise your bad cholesterol (LDL) while they lower your good cholesterol (HDL) levels. Zombies increase your risk of stroke and heart disease. Stay away from their hidden nights of living dead, please.

I *don't* advocate that you transform into a label-reading fanatic at the food market or obsess in your kitchen about an occasional snack of popcorn that has some less-than-good fats. Yet, *please* check your foods' breakouts of fats, plus salts, preservatives, and the type of carbohydrates within the package or box. Your lifespan depends on that. The list goes on…

Remember that fiber is a component of healthy carbohydrates as one of your macronutrients. As a supplemental takeaway, please avoid "cured" meats. The preservative process with sodium nitrates does the *opposite* of curing cancer! It converts to *nitrosamine*, a known carcinogen.[87] And please think twice before adding monosodium glutamates as your flavor enhancers. Please recognize surrogate names for simple, high-glycemic-index sugars too. Have you seen these pseudonym syrups when playing Sherlock Holmes?

- Maize syrup
- Glucose syrup – some evil HFCS may actually be processed from glucose.

- Tapioca syrup
- Crystalline fructose
- Dahlia syrup.

It takes more than "just the fats" and syrupy smarts to be a culinary student of your endeavor.

FLEX ALERT #26:

You want and need the "right" fats in your lifestyle diet. Not too little, not too much. And you don't need odorous fish oil to boost your absorbed levels of Omega-3 fatty acids.

Hemp seeds and chia seeds are two alternate sources of "heart healthy" Omega-3 fatty acids, plus they provide high-fiber content. In moderation, these seeds are very good boosters for strong GenX individuals without causing gut issues in most folks. Free-range eggs can be boosted for higher Omega-3 content too because those hens eat flaxseed-supplemented diets.

- Remember that high Omega-3s are heart-healthy good, while high Omega-6 fatty acid levels are generally not. As an example, wild salmon is quite high in Omega-3s, while tilapia is high in Omega-6 fatty acids.

Scientists tell us that foods with a high ratio of Omega-6 to Omega-3 are *not* good for heart health. A ratio of over 4:1 is deemed to be high and unhealthy due to pro-inflammatory responses that are made by your body. (Note that I flipped the Omegas fraction here. I cited a healthy 1:4 guideline of Omega 3 to Omega 6 earlier.) Let's revisit another bit of good and not-so-good nutrition.

"GOOD" NITRATES

Good nitrates for performance are quite different from the cancer-promoting nitrates of processed or cured meats (like some bacon or cold cuts). A good nitrogen compound, aka nitrate, truly benefits your athlete within:

> "nitrate, which is abundant in green leafy vegetables
> and roots, has ... effects that include a reduction in
> blood pressure, modification of platelet aggregation
> and increases in limb blood flow."[88]

More flow, less pressure, all great.

Beets, spinach, and kale are also natural sources of nitrates that your kidneys process into nitric oxide (with a chemical symbol of NO). Watermelon and cucumbers are fine sources of a nonessential amino acid called L-Citrulline that promotes nitric oxide production in your body too. (This is just one nitrogen molecule short of being nitrous oxide—the dentist's *laughing gas*.) Yet, this nitric "Doctor NO" is no laughing matter. In fact, Dr. NO is so important that the 1998 Nobel Prize in Medicine was awarded to three researchers who discovered how "NO" relaxes blood vessels and cues one's cardiovascular system. Honest.

Yes, NO is a fat-soluble gas that may improve your bodily immune defenses. NO helps increase blood flow when metabolic demands are high, as found in "red zone" sessions of weight training or in TABATA high-intensity interval training (HIIT) protocols. Nitric oxide has been seriously studied as an ergogenic aid since 2007. Believe it or not, your nose can enable your body's temporal production of the NO gas.

THE NOSE KNOWS.

After nasal inhalations, your sinuses produce NO to fight harmful bacteria and viruses (like COVID-19). But more, your nasal inhalations complement the main production of transitory NO gas by your kidneys to help regulate blood pressure. Yup! Plus, the vasodilation role of bodily NO signals can help you stay strong to save—particularly in your endurance work or stamina exercises.

Researchers suggest that small doses of nitrates taken over several days (either plant-based or supplemental NO) *may* increase your fast twitch (Type II) muscle activation, and they appear to boost your maximal power output.

The boost period of NO for activation or power generation is only about six hours. Me? I take L-citrulline gel capsules daily to help release NO. I eat beets and spinach and drink tomato juice quite often.

SUPER NATURAL

Since I'm writing about foods with Vitamin (P) for NO production, I share my operational definition of a *superfood*. A superfood is a plant-based product that reduces inflammation in your or my system, microbiome, or gut. Superfoods can be roots, leafy green vegetables, legumes, alliums (like onions or leeks), or mushrooms, or herbs and spices. Be colorful, not drab in your approach to "clean" eating.

- Eat supernaturally with regular rainbow-colored meals to offset ROS.

Yes, superfoods are natural ergogenics that improve your physical bank and downaged health span. They lower inflammation or pain from ADL or resistance training. Yes, there will be times when anti-inflammatory foods are *not* quite enough to address your inflammation or pain. This is a great GenX fact of life. Here comes another important acronym for your recognition – NSAID.

NSAID

Aspirin, Tylenol™, Aleve™, and Cipro™ are common over the counter or prescription "pain killers" that are classified as NSAIDs.

The NSAID acronym stands for a non-steroidal anti-inflammatory *drug*. Note my italicized emphasis on the term *drug*, which is important. I hope and pray that you can avert drug-taking and polypharmacy when alternatives exist. And they do, despite Madison Avenue marketing blitzes for "safe" NSAIDs.

A retired MD shared with me that human bodies can take care of most health issues without a doctor's call or prescribed drugs. Your body can handle about ~80 percent of what life puts in the way of your healthy journey.

Think about that when you develop episodic pains from work or exercise, please. Think about mindful breathing and your cognitive tricks as two alternative to popping expensive generic or brand name drugs. Let's face this reality: these NSAIDs are readily available in America's multi-billion-dollar market, with annual growth rates of 5 percent.[89]

It is evident that Madison Avenue and "Big Pharma" want you to have these painkillers on your shelf and in your gym bag. Sure, NSAIDs are widely used to relieve pain, reduce inflammation, and bring down a person's high temperature. Drugs should not be taken lightly in my book.

When I contracted COVID-19 recently, a nice GP in Athenry Ireland advised me to rest, get fresh air, and take "Tylenol" as needed to get my temperature back to normal. No PAXLOVID™, nothing prescriptive … *Ireland is a great spot to self-isolate from a SARS virus, by the way.* This practical Doc appreciated how strong bodies can counter cytokine storms and mentioned that side effects of some COVID drugs are worse than the symptoms when you are not a high-risk individual. Let me shift from the fields of Athenry to the playing fields where NSAID use might be considered.

Endurance and ultra-endurance athletes *may* get a boost from their timely downing of a NSAID. I have a great GenX rowing buddy who is also a nut for ultra-endurance events like the daunting Leadville race series held in the Colorado Rockies. He *did* get an ergogenic boost from careful doses of a NSAID on his sixth and successful attempt. Well done, Jim!

I do not know of any ergogenic boost from a NSAID for weightlifting, other than for pain reduction. Next, here are some "drug" derivatives or alternatives that you might cautiously consider for inflammation, discomfort, or pain...

TOPICAL SUBSTANCES

CBD: Non-hallucinogenic cannabidiol (CBD) ointments, patches, or oils can address anxiety and possibly lessen some chronic pains of an athlete. When the psychoactive compound of cannabis (THC) is removed to make "safe" CBD products, the concern of drug highs is lessened or removed. As with many ergogenics, CBD is touted for many nonverified treatments and cures. CBD is not, to date, a CRAAP-tested[1] performance enhancer, unless your pre-event anxieties are high. I have no personal experiences with CBD, so I leave you to make your own decision about safe CBD use. Make a note that placebos can be effective, so one's MBA studies will find ironies and hard to explain facts.

GROOVY

Well, the far-out sixties of Timothy Leary were long, long ago. Some endurance athletes now assert that *psylocibin* (magic mushrooms) alters their minds' perceptions of discomfort or pain. I suggest you wait for credible clinical tests before trying psychedelics in hopes of performance gains in endurance events. Granted, I have little doubt

---

[1] CRAAP-tested means that a source is: current, relevant, authoritative, accurate, and published.

that psychedelics can dampen effects of brain disorders like veterans' post-traumatic stress disorders (PTSD) from combat shock. Yet, consider your jury still out on ergogenic use. Plus, I have not read any credible research articles about psychedelics as strength ergogenics.

YOU'VE READ THIS BEFORE

More research is needed to understand how CBD, psychedelics and other substances impact athletic performance, health, or other exercise-training outcomes.

As I mentioned, athletes may need supplements in their clean diets because of their training loads. Ladies – I will defer discussion of potential female supplements until I co-author a sequel with a female athlete who can also speak from her experiences.

Gents – it may be helpful for you to consider what I consciously take in my 70s to keep thriving and striving as a masters athlete. Now, some of these entries are worthy of female attention, too.

You previously read about my green tea and coffee drinks, my AREDS2 vitamin use, and my L-Citrulline supplementation to help produce NO. I may also use melatonin if travel or demands of life challenge my restorative sleep patterns.

I supplement natural sunlight with Vitamin D3, despite living in sunny Southern California.

I take Biotin (Vitamin B-7) which I believe helps support collagen production– the most prevalent protein in my body.

My Dermatologist suggests I take Vitamin B-3 (Niacinamide) to potentially reduce pre-cancerous skin damage called actinic keratoses. My complexion and genetics make me a very regular guest of dermatologists, so I took this suggestion seriously. Thus B-3 may help at a price that I can afford.

I sense that frankincense, a resin from Boswellia trees, *may* modify bodily discomfort and pain. Heck, frankincense was good enough to be a gift of the Magi, and there are no known side effects. Hence, I choose to give it an experimental go *without* scientific proof. My go is still a' goin.

I am currently trying berberine, which is sometimes called "nature's OZEMPIC™." *No*, I didn't try berberine because it is popular and trending on social media. My third party-tested berberine also has anti-inflammatory cinnamon in it. I don't take prescription drugs that might interact with berberine, and my gut does not seem disturbed by the quantity I take. I am not taking it for weight loss. Yet, it just might help improve my *insulin sensitivity* as I age.

I don't take little blue pills for libido. Yet I do more than dabble with a traditional medicine root extract from Asia named Tong kat Ali that translates to "Ali's walking stick." I am intrigued by its bioactive chemicals. Likewise, I note small western research studies that suggest this *walking stick*, in small doses, may enhance muscle development and reduce stress. I am monitoring my intake for side effects, and as I don't take any prescription drugs, side effects are not an issue.

My GP is aware that I take saw palmetto pills to address my slight benign prostate enlargement from aging. As I sleep through nights without waking for bladder relief, this saw palmetto is a low-risk preventative for me. I reinforce that my Doctor is aware of this "OTC" use and that I monitor for gut issues or side effects with other ergogenics or nutrients.

Though this list is already long, I add a "well tolerated" traditional adaptogen, ashwagandha, as another supplement that is worthy of consideration. I consider it worthy as my chosen brand is third party-tested and it seems to assist me in my vigorous lifestyle and quest for restorative sleep. I also like my ashwagandha supplement's combination with ginger and turmeric for added anti-inflammatory bennies.

Ashwagandha is one of many supplements that *hasn't* been scrutinized in long-term research studies (yet.) You just might find that a ~ 225 mg daily dose can, over time, improve sexual function for both genders, and reduce brain fog. Not bad at all, in my book.

Yes, some folks may have side effects in the gut. Some folks should not take ashwagandha, like breast feeding moms, some with auto-immune disorders, or if they are taking certain prescription medications.

Speaking of other supplements, two A-to-Z examples are added for your final consideration of supplements from nature. Yup, I take both, with my Doctor's awareness. Bottom line? I ingest a dozen supplements regularly, yet I do it prudently and with my MD's awareness.

ASTAXANTHIN

A powerful carotenoid, astaxanthin, is both a natural source and supplemental antioxidant that can potentially improve lifespans.[90] Wild salmon that ingest certain invertebrate organisms—like krill or algae—keep astaxanthin in the human food chain. Conversely, one can safely take astaxanthin supplements (without a fishy smell or burping of fish oil) to reap most of the *foodborne* benefits of antioxidant astaxanthin.

Absorbed astaxanthin increases glucose intake by your skeletal muscles and improves your insulin sensitivity. Both roles can be very good boosts, at least in lower mammal research studies. Bear in mind that credible clinical trials for life-extending properties predominate in *mice,* not in *humans.*

With that note, I offer that I eat plenty of wild salmon, and I do take supplemental astaxanthin capsules. I think of this supplement as part of my affordable life insurance. Now, zoom to the other end of our alphabet for a final anti-inflammatory booster.

ZEAXANTHIN

The carotenoid zeaxanthin is a fat-soluble antioxidant. (Lutein and zeaxanthin are the two main carotenoids for eye health.) In plain sight, zeaxanthin plays a key role in your good vision and eye health.

Plus, it is known to reduce your risk of vision loss from macular degeneration.

Eggs and leafy green vegetables are great natural sources of this carotenoid. Yet many people like me do *not* leave eye health to chickens and broccoli alone. As you read earlier, I hedge my inflammation-fighting bet for eye health with daily AREDS2 supplements. In your physical banking, as in fiscal banking for nest eggs, hedge funds and prudent bets just may work for you. However, there will be a day when your bank is temporarily under-performing.

SAY WHAT? A MASTERS ATHLETE WILL UNDER-PERFORM.

I bet you two nickels that a great GenX will develop marginal deficiencies at some point from an *over*training condition.

Other than my OURA™ fitness ring, which you will soon read about, my sainted wife serves as the canary in coalmine alert for my overtraining. "You are a bit snippy" or "you fell asleep after dinner" are two of her canary songs directed at me...

When you over-train, a marginal deficiency of one or more micronutrients may occur. And your restorative sleep suffers. And you may find yourself on a performance plateau.

Both sickness and over-training involve inflammation. *You definitely want to avoid sickness from training too hard for too long.* Remember that muscular inflammation is both your friend and your foe. When too much inflammation arises from over-training, absorbing a carotenoid or a good fatty acid can naturally help, yet not immediately. Remember what Tour de France riders take during their assuredly overtrained rides? Vitamin D3.

Remember that our government calls its micronutrient guidelines "minimum daily requirements (MDRs)" for good reason. If you are sick, working your metabolism greatly, or are over-trained, a MDR may be *in*adequate for health span. Yet, also remember that too much of a good micro is *not* always wonderful.

Iron is one of those "too much" mineral candidates, particularly for male GenX. And another...As a fat-soluble vitamin, E can potentially stockpile to excess in your corpus. Vitamins A, D, E, and K are fat-soluble. Water-soluble vitamins, like the B series and C, do not hang around. If taken in excess, your gut may rebel with these water-soluble vitamins, and your urine becomes a wee bit pricey. So, what is my experienced "bet" and recommendation for your proper micro-nutrition in normal training conditions?

YOU BETCHA

I prudently take key micronutrients to supplement my nutritional levels *beyond* what our government labels as daily guidelines. Guidelines are just guidelines for the average American, and I am *not* average. Neither are you as a great GenX.

I cautiously ingest and absorb what seems to work for me. Magnesium is one of my key examples. The harder I train in my periodizations, the more I need my "right" micro-deposits of magnesium and the more Epsom salt soaks I take. You betcha... the more you know, the better you can overcome those marginal deficiencies, as a Tour de France rider or as you with your $10 Million physical bank.

I'll add an interesting application of Vitamin C which I recently adopted. Why? As you and I age, our skin loses its elasticity (unless you are a blessed Hollywood starlet.) Yes, a third-party tested vitamin C serum, in combination with 3 well-documented skin compounds – hyaluronic acid, salicylic acid, and niacinamide retinol – *can* counter skin-aging for you.

I also find that "my" serum is far less costly than many "wonder treatments" you can find on shelves or on-line. A great and studious GenX can find *affordable and effective* skin treatments that do help with aesthetic appeal. As the largest organ in your body by area, your skin merits great serums, in my opinion and experience. This is a perfectly good time to consider Father or Mother Time and even that platitude about an early bird and worms.

SUBCHAPTER 2—TIMING IS ALMOST EVERYTHING

I endorse *When? The Scientific Secrets of Perfect Timing*, by Daniel Pink in 2018, as another book to "chew and digest thoroughly", as Francis Bacon suggested.

Why? Early birds generally catch the worms. Night hawks generally catch whatever they can. Third birds – well – I am sure that they catch their meals too. No one of these 3 types of "birds" is inherently better or worse than the others. Thus, it is smart to understand all three chronotypes, three...

Are you a morning lark or a night hawk or a third bird? (A third bird is someone inclined to wake between eight and ten on a typical morning). This query is relative, rather than absolute, as you may well be a hybrid chronotype or a variable feathered friend.

Dan Pink suggests, as do I, that you try the Munich Chronotype Questionnaire (MCTQ) to assess your internal clock. *Why not give this questionnaire a try?* You can easily find a free copy of this MCTQ online.

Yes, you can embrace and optimize your daily and nightly patterns and preferences. Get rhythm on your side—daily—to stay strong to save.

Granted, Pink's colorful and credible account of timing gone right and wrong deals with more than strength workouts.

Yet, you will enjoy dog-earing and highlighting key concepts for athletic achievement as you consider his authored content of *When?* I guarantee that you will "sync" up and use your own scientific clock in helpful, rhythmic ways. Chrono-what?

CIRCADIAN RHYTHMS

A chronotype is your natural internal clock in contrast to the twenty-four-hour external clock of waking and sleeping imposed by your work, travel, and environment.

In modern life, chronotypes are internal wake-sleep patterns that conform or contrast with natural or artificial light. I hope that you have a natural rhythm, as being in a sleep-deprived state is un-natural and certainly is *not* fun at all. I commend to you the credible resources of our national Sleep Foundation, as well as Daniel Pink's timely book.

Let's also consider timed milestones in a strength periodization, or in macro cycles of achievement. Why? A great GenX should have project manager skills as well F.I.T.T. skills.

Think about the choice of, and milestone results from:

- starting,
- midpoint or halftime, and
- ending timestamps

of your chosen endeavor.

When you plan your athletic endeavors, you want to make that endeavor's midpoint a spark rather than a sputter. Right? Your midpoints (or half times) are wonderful points to reassess, recalibrate, and get it on for the second half. Your macro cycle end points are perfect times to reflect and document your lessons learned. Then, that endpoint serves as a base camp for your next ascent.

Let's assess how chrono typing and timing can affect your project-managed strengths for micro- and meso-cycles of periodization.

MORNING METAL?

When you choose to weightlift may be necessitated by your work and/ or family schedules. Whether you choose, or whether you need to get that resistance training session in before noon *does* matter.

Recall this key differentiation from chapter 2 of Strong to Save: cell growth processes are "anabolic," while cell teardown processes that atrophy your sarcomeres are "catabolic."

Do you lift in morning times without breaking the fast to maintain or "tone" (meaning many repetitions done with relatively light loading)? If so, you can probably stay in an anabolic or building state, rather than experience an unwanted tear-down, catabolic state. Anabolism versus catabolism is a complicated, yet important point for your timely and strong GenX efforts.

- Attempts at high volume and intensity in strength training, before you refuel, can deplete your muscle stores and tear-down what you've tried to build up. Granted, this approach may help you shed a little fat, or it may instead deplete your muscles. I believe that you can effectively lift in fasted states and "satisfice" strength and fat loss goals. Yet, this is difficult. Be careful of your performance goals and know your body's response to fasted weight workouts.

Do not act like a slow or fast Sisyphus. Remember that poor legend, Sisyphus? He was doomed to push a rock up the steep hill, then to watch it roll back down for his endless do-overs. A great GenX adopts different tactics than did Sisyphus.

BREAK THE FAST?

A notable percentage of trained and experienced CrossFit athletes carefully deploy intermittent fasting and exercise (IFE), and so can you. This is true if a great GenX chooses to pack two complementary workouts in for a day. Rowers like me practice at low- to mid- intensity in predawn and early times of day when we are "*hangry*." Some folks call such a low intensity routine "fat burning," which is true yet is also oversimplified.

Remember that your daily energy equation is the summation of waves of hormonal and chemical processes, coupled with variances of high and low energy demands. Those internal, clocked processes are based on restorative states, replenishment of glucose and glycogen, and more.

Me? I do *not* "lift heavy" in a fasted state in morning time. I often do bodyweight exercises when fasted. And I invest these early workout times to bank my stamina, stability, and flexibility. As a (mostly) morning lark, I invest a majority of my A.M. training time (yup – up to 75%-80%) in steady-state, low-intensity efforts. My sweaty work is done in a crew shell, on a trail by dawn's early light, or on a stationary cycle for 60 to 90 minutes.

If I do high volume or intense weight lifting before noon, I ensure that I eat a mini meal about an hour prior. That fast-breaker meal includes protein and carbohydrates because I don't want to be self-defeating.

Again, if you tap too much energy in the wrong way at the wrong time, you likely catabolize your muscles, and that is *not* good.

Know that your body is "wired" to tap muscle as a source of bodily fuel *before* white fat is chosen as a source of energy. Yup. It is millennia of human survival at work, so neither you nor I can (currently) change that ... Rather, try to factor *how* you exercise *when* you exercise to be in anabolic states, naturally.

AFTERNOON DELIGHT

Consider that many national and world or Olympic records are set in afternoon settings. Yet, resistance exercise done *too* close to your bedtime *isn't* wonderful. Morning times through early evening periods are the best times to elevate your heart rate with stamina or strength activities. For most of us, exercising too close to slumber time can defer or defeat our intended drowsiness and deep sleep. Why? Excess post-exercise oxygen consumption (EPOC), a.k.a. "afterburn," with an accompanying elevated heart rate, adversely affects your normal unwinding and pre-sleep efforts.

DAILY DOUBLES?

One emergent phenomenon (2023) is that "everyday exercisers" are joining triathletes, elite Masters performers, and professional athletes by doubling down on some days of each week.

I often get sweaty and sore from *daily doubles* because I need the exercise volume in some of my periodizations. Others get in twice as nice workouts of short durations in a day as that tempo fits their lifestyle.

If I was to add a postscript to Daniel Pink's fine work, *When*, this is what it would be:

Make two-a-day workouts an optional piece of your great gameplan.

Balance quantity and quality. Be wary of over-training. Ask yourself, is today a better day to rest and recover? And space your double-down workouts at least 5 hours apart.

It is a great time to wind up this sub-chapter.

SUMMARY

Your conscious timing of training and supportive sustenance isn't everything, yet it is far more than nuttin'. Take advantage of your daily time passages. You perform at your best when you leverage the variable waves of your very own daily energy processes.

Stay naturally anabolic to build your H&S or power capacity. Fat-burn in the morning and know how to leverage IFE. Pursue your strong personal bests in the afternoon when you are locked and loaded with fuel to build up your VITA. Never discount or forget that restorative sleep is a vital part of your chronotype and ultimately of your strong performance. Do not misplace your Swiss army utility tool...*sleep*.

SUBCHAPTER 3—MIMIC MORPHEUS

Matthew Walker, PhD, neuroscientist, and sleep researcher at UC Berkley, tells us, "Sleep is the Swiss army knife of health. When sleep is deficient, there is sickness and disease. And when sleep is abundant, there is vitality and health."[91] See Figure 8.2.

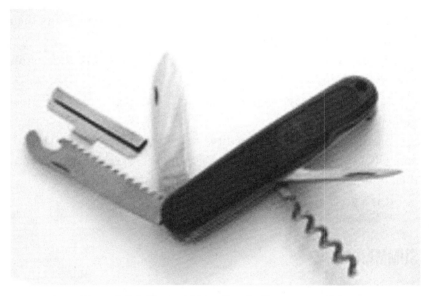

Figure 8.2 A Physical Metaphor for Restorative Sleep

I just know that you chose vitality and health over sickness and disease for your journey. Now, let's examine what role restorative sleep plays for vitality and health. Could there be something mythical about that sleep role?

Yes, you *can* convincingly cheat death for a spell, like the mythical Greek character, Morpheus. You can dazzle others like the character Morpheus in *The Matrix* movie series. Soak that in for a minute.

- You can cheat death and gain extra years with restful sleep as your utility knife.

This is my lone suggestion to cheat in your game of life. Why is cheating good in this case?

Because *one-third* of all people in GenX, both males and postmenopausal females, have diagnosed or *un*diagnosed sleep disorders! *Oy*. Imagine how sleep deprivation dulls your own Swiss army knife.

Some of these sleep problems or disorders, like obstructive sleep apnea (OSA) can be life-threatening. I confidently state that some sleep disorders can be accommodated. I am living proof of that.

PROOF POSITIVE

Years ago, my wonderful wife timed my nighttime breath stoppages at sixty-plus seconds. Back then, I also caught myself dozing on my afternoon forty-five-minute commutes. I was also prone to nodding off at late night parties.

My breath stoppages, highway scares, and party doze-offs were tipping points to get medical help. I didn't smoke, except for a rare celebratory Cubano. I didn't drink alcohol to excess. I wasn't overweight. I had, and have, a lean 16¾ inch neck. I am lucky that I never faced post-traumatic stress disorder (PTSD).

Not one of these top causes of OSA was my sleep issue. Rather, my relaxed soft palate triggered "moderate" OSA, and that coulda killed me. Honest – *Sleep apnea is a killer.* I now don my CPAP mask nightly to gain restful sleep and stay alive longer. (CPAP is shorthand for a continuous positive airway pressure machine) My prescribed CPAP chooses the right pressure to stimulate my "regular," *non*-apnea breathing for sleep.

Yes, there are surgical techniques and dental appliances that may help some folks address their sleep apnea. If you are diagnosed – pick a remedial approach and stick with it for your life and breath. I kid you not. As a testimony, I find that the comfort of CPAP masks is becoming less of an excuse for non-users as they get smaller, lighter, and more comfortable.

Get over any hassle, folks. *Do not* traverse that river called *"de nial."* A degree of white machine noise is preferable to high-decibel disturbing snores, right? To be clear on that aspect, a snorer may not have apnea, yet a person with apnea likely snores, and often when his or her body reacts to lack of oxygen.

I love my improved, restorative deep sleep with that CPAP. Why? I am very partial to *stayin' alive, stayin' alive.* My nightly restorative processes release natural human growth hormones, restore my noggin's clear thinking, and promote muscular repair after my workouts and activity.

As for you, ask not to live in denial, and do not avoid professional help for something so precious as your sleep. Ladies—note that you may suffer OSA after menopause at similar rates to gentlemen. *No* GenX should be sleepless in Spokane, Seattle, or Shakopee. It is time for three WIFMs to mimic Morpheus.

THREE SLEEPLESS FACTS OF LIFE:

1. Less sleep equates to less caloric burn for your basic metabolic rate.
2. Less quality sleep means less cleansing of your brain circuitry.
3. Less sleep means less stamina and strength to get it on and keep it on. *Oy vey.*

Let's agree on what sleep is, thanks to *Webster's* or dictionary.com. Sleep is

"a naturally occurring, reversible, periodic and recurring state in which consciousness and muscular activity is temporarily suspended or diminished, and responsiveness to outside stimuli is reduced."[92]

Check, Morpheus.

REALITY CHECK

Right, the word morphine stems from that sleepy Greek figure's name, Morpheus. Too few of us will sleep like babies tonight, even if you or I say *Morpheus*. Wouldn't it be nice to sleep long and hard like that romantic cherub, without a care in the world?

Check this: you decompress as your brain, endocrine system, and gut generate your happy hormones with restorative sleep. However:

- Some ladies in GenX endure exhausting hot flashes.
- The parental guardian in you is worried about your adult kids' careers and their little ones.
- You get restless legs or cramps.

WHY, WHY, SIX HUNDRED TIMES WHY

Sara Gottfried, MD, a respected sleep guru, offers this genetic wakeup call:

"Sleep governs over six hundred genes—weight loss genes ... and genes that predict your risk of Alzheimer's disease."[93]

The National Institutes of Health reports, "When our biological clock is disrupted, it can cause sleep disorders and other problems, like *obesity, depression, heart disease, high blood pressure and diabetes.* Researchers ... have found a new link between a circadian clock gene called nocturnin and obesity."[94]

Further, inadequate sleep chemically raises levels of ghrelin, that darned hormone that makes you feel hungry. By now, the importance of restorative sleep should be catching your full attention.

You need about seven to eight hours of sleep per night to fit into your jeans and to repair, restore, and rebuild your sarcomeres after you weight train. What are some restful resources for your study efforts? One resource is our National Sleep Foundation that addresses wonderful *whys* or WIFMs for restful sleep.

✓ Do check out www.thensf.org/.[95] Better restorative sleep beats counting sheep or being drunk, and that is the truth. A non-profit website by the American Lung Association, www.lung.org, reinforces the importance of your vital lung capacity and offers a platitude to remember, "a good day begins with a good night's sleep."

FLEX ALERT #27:

Sleep is not overrated! Eighteen hours *without* sleep is tantamount to a blood alcohol reading near 0.05 percent for impaired driving.

You don't want a highway patrolman to pull you over for being tipsy from either sleep deprivation or friendly spirits imbibed in a pub. You do want help, however, to gain something so vital for strength.

SLEEP AIDS

There are many scientific reasons to get your restorative sleep. And there are many, many methods that supposedly, possibly, or probably aid in your sleep. Trust them, perhaps, yet verify 'em fer sure. It depends on what works for you. Help with sleep disorders may even come from federally funded resources.

HI, I'M FROM THE GOVERNMENT, AND I'M HERE TO HELP

Here are three federal "wake-up" calls from *Your Guide to Healthy Sleep*, that is distributed by the National Institutes of Health:

1. "A chronic lack of sleep increases your risk of obesity, diabetes, cardiovascular disease, and infections."

2. "Because of your body's internal processes, you *can't* adapt to getting less sleep than your body needs."[96] *Please read this number 2 again!*
3. "We sleep two hours less than Americans did a century ago."

If your body needs sleep, you cannot adapt or do without it! Pull an all-nighter and you may get pulled over! This sleep guide *is* federal tax dollars put to good, preventative use.

Also, the Centers for Disease Control and Prevention states that adults sleeping less than seven hours per night have an *increased* risk of several diseases, including CVD.[97] And, as CVD is the largest cause of illness and death for American adults, I'm all aboard the Ben Franklin sleep train for worthy ounces of prevention. How about you?

The federal sleep guide also provides a fine summary of what our brains do while we are asleep.

POUNDAGE

Your brain is *working overtime* while the rest of your body is in your nightly slumber stages. Well-documented studies record that our brains burn calories through our sleep time as much as a 35- to 75-watt light bulb would. *Wanna lose weight?* Sleep!

If you have an average metabolic rate and sleep soundly for seven hours, that's about 450 dietary calories that are "brain burned." That's correct. One-quarter to one-third of your resting metabolism is from sleep expenditures. And expensed for great causes—like restoration, cleansing, and recovery. *Cleansing?* Right.

Our brains are fascinating in many ways. One fact is that our noggins do not have a normal "plumbing" (i.e., a lymphatic) system like the rest of your body. If you *don't* sleep adequately or exercise properly, your brain's waste-disposal system cannot complete its critical cleansing role to keep you from exhaustion.

SLEEP ZOMBIES

Deprivation is *not* a good thing to experience or sustain. Physical dangers or harm and certainly grouchiness will result from missed opportunities to restore and recharge your mind and body. Sure, we hear about individuals in Navy SEAL hell week, and in other-worldly challenges, when personnel can and do press on, like zombies.

Ultra-endurance events, like extreme Mudder events or the six-day, 140-mile trans-Sahara foot race, or those Badlands 135-mile ultramarathons (which start in Death Valley, California, each July), are very good for zombie Guinness World Records.

Yet these overachieving and sleep-deprived participants experience "awful afters" as they face many weeks of recovery. Exemplar: a gent who set the world record for distance covered in 24 hours on a treadmill almost died from his internal organs shutdown. And you could be living a lifetime of "awful afters" by being deprived of sleep on a nightly basis over the years.

You can't become or remain a great GenX if you can't cope and mimic Morpheus.

WHAT ABOUT NAPS?

Snoozing under the right conditions after caffeine is taken, for what Dan Pink calls a nappucino in *When*, can *improve* performances after noon. Yup! And it works very nicely for me.

Here's the nappucino hack:

- ✓ drink your preferred caffeinated beverage,
- ✓ hit the rocking chair or couch or put your head down on your workplace desk,
- ✓ tune out for a timed twenty minutes.

Why? Your caffeine boost begins in about that same twenty minutes as your shuteye. Then splash some water on your happy mug and restfully carry on with your chronotype day.

Your catch-up naps or snoozes, like "sleeping-in" routines on weekends or special days, are great indeed. These siestas address short-term sleep shortages that are bad, bad in many, many ways. Who hasn't awakened feeling refreshed after a twenty-minute siesta? Put a little caffeinated zip in this equation and you are good to go.

Note the approximate limit for a good nap—*twenty* minutes. Why? After taking a half-hour nap or longer, you may have trouble shaking away your cognitive cobwebs, and this may impede that night's critical sleep. So, how are stress and sleep related?

SLEEP AND STRESS SIDEBARS

Alcohol (with a long half-life in your body) lifts cortisol levels, which may contribute to heart-thumping awakenings in your wee morning hours. Your adrenal cortisol adversely impacts your parasympathetic feed-and-restore rhythms. These are healthy rhythms that would otherwise help you get ready for your next strength regimen.

- Cortisol is a fat-related hormone, that is *bad* when it is stays chronically high from stressors.

Sure, some folks are luckier than others with their handling of caffeine and alcohol. Thus, their cortisol doesn't spike or persist. Some, like me, find that certain types of alcohol cause nighttime waking impacts and cortisol bumps that are greater than other types. I wish it wasn't so, yet red wines may cause my 3 a.m. heart-thumpin' reveilles. I also find, by the way, that summertime iced tea can wire me up more than my preferred social stimulant, coffee.

- Know your sense-and-respond reactions to natural stimulants and depressants—like caffeine and alcohol.

Cortisol and adrenal stress responses are *not* your strong-to-save allies, except in danger zones.

Exceptions to our routines, perhaps holidays, special late-night parties, late-evening airport pickups, or time zone travels are facts of modern life. In my case, teaching adult learners at night is an exception to my routine. I situationally get paid to be alert on my feet at 10:00 p.m., so I may drink "leaded" coffee before or in class on my teaching nights. I'm blessed that I can generally fall asleep and remain that way after I get home from those night classes. And I go to sleep without a nightcap. Right, every athlete (and in my case, adjunct professor) has unique sleep patterns and perturbations. Know yours as a student or professor of your endeavors.

It is now time to laud females of GenX that deal directly with menopause (and childbirth.) In a spirit of equality, I also cite challenges of manopause.

Ladies, please take the enlightening quiz in Dr. Sara Gottfried's book, *The Hormone Cure*.[98] Yes, there *are* natural alternatives to polypharmacy that can aid your better sleep habits.

I laud today's publicity for menopause and perimenopause after being hush-hush since Victorian days. When Oprah Winfrey and Michelle Obama speak openly about female midlife realities and encourage a social network of menopause parties, life can only get better.

LISTEN UP, GUYS.

Restorative sleep is a natural counter for androgen deficiency in the aging male (ADAM) and "*manopause*" hassles for men. Please take what is known as the Saint Louis quiz of ten questions to assess your vital, manly hormones, particularly "T". Go to this credible Nature website: https://www.nature.com/articles/ijir200935.

Perhaps one percent of GenX males experience manopause – maybe less or may be more. These are androgen deficient symptoms that can be overcome after crossing that certain river starting with the letter "d"…

- ED
- Fatigue
- Advancing sarcopenia
- Increasing body fat and central obesity
- Decrease in bone mass
- Mood changes
- Disturbed sleep and
- Anxiety or depression.

None of the ADAM symptoms are good for either Adam or his Eve. And, sooner or later, an older GenX may see a trend toward a higher St. Louis score. Guys – don't let that happen without a fight.

Both genders need to take this reminder for your sleep bank: You **need** sleep to optimize your bodily production of:

- ✓ Testosterone
- ✓ Serotonin as your reward and motivation neurotransmitter
- ✓ Dopamine as your mind and body's anti-depressant and mood stabilizer. Yes, exercise also boosts dopamine levels.

When serotonin and dopamine raise, cortisol drops. All you need is sleep (and exercise). Add love if you like the lyrics of one Beatles song. Next, how about your physical sleep aids?

PILLOW TALK

Cervical pillows, oxygen pillows, apnea pillows, oh my. Buyers must beware of much Madison Avenue hype about costly sleep "solutions." Yet don't rule out affordable pillows that promote spinal stability, good breathing, and deep sleep. And don't forget to find that ideal mattress to provide the best spinal alignment for your sleeping partner (if applicable) and for you.

Should you want an eerie feeling, you can check the weight of dust mites and excreta that accumulate in older mattresses and mattress pads. I kid you not!

Swap out that oldie mattress or pad and get the best possible mattress cover to keep mites out. These covers are worth your investment. Take your position, please.

SLEEP HABITS

We are sleepers of habit. So, my suggestion that you try a varied sleep position may go over like a lead balloon. I can only offer that I became a mixed back and side sleeper after my spinal fusion surgery. I was formerly a regal snoozer and sleeper: meaning face upward and flat on my back. I'm suggesting that by trying different positions, you might learn something and possibly get better sleep.

Researchers from Johns Hopkins suggest that sleep positions can affect specific conditions such as acid reflux, back and neck pain, snoring, and apnea.[99] Don't let detractors like these affect your strength endeavors, please. Now, do you wear PJs?

SLEEPWEAR OR NOT

I don't gain favor with nightgown and pajama retailers by suggesting that you might sleep with "nothing on at all." Yet, health professionals and I can share healthy reasons why sleeping without PJs is good, or at least worth a proverbial try.

Why not try it, if you haven't? You (and your human sleep partner) may like it. And you just might be healthier too, even in fall and winter. I mentioned *human*, as there isn't a ton of research suggesting that a furry friend who shares your bed might improve your deep sleep, whatever you wear or don't.

TIM AND I

Author and podcaster Tim Ferriss offers his tips to unwind before evening sleep in *Tools of Titans*[99]. I'll share just one:

- He invests five to ten minutes before his lights out time to get his to-do list off his mind, which also drops his cortisol level a bit.

How do I enhance restorative sleep, even when challenged by stresses and strains of my life?

- Warm Epsom salt baths, finished ninety minutes before my own "taps."

We absorb magnesium through our pores and actually burn a few calories when immersed and perspiring in a sauna or bathtub. However, my own heart rate elevates when in a sauna hot tub, so I need some cool-down time, like 90 minutes, before calling it a night.

I find it both interesting and effective that a cool shower can have the same sleepy effects as that warm soothing bath, provided that a shower is finished sixty to ninety minutes before you turn out your lights.

My sleep professional once suggested that I try a prescription "lifeline" when I was mentally *wired* about a big workplace commitment. I tried one-half of a tiny (prescription) Ambien tablet under my tongue for those episodic, restless nights of stress. Ambien seemed to work, and I only took it situationally.

I hope that you can sense and appreciate my nature-first, prescription-second approach for a strong-to-save lifestyle. Sleep is so critical, however, that I give a tacit thumbs-up for "some" drugs like Ambien when used sparingly. Nature, you say.

MELLOWING MELATONIN

Our "Paleo" forbearers could generate plenty of *natural* melatonin by sleeping many more hours than we do today. After singing around their campfires and staring at starry nights, they had no problem getting twelve hours of circadian sleep. The only reliable light they had was sunlight, so their circadian dark times enabled melatonin production in buckets.

What happened since the Industrial Revolution? Nowadays, city and office lights that never dim (unless there is a blackout), your extensive screen times plus artificial lights, and third-bird or nighthawk work schedules mess with your natural melatonin processes.

When I travel across time zones by air, or if I train quite hard on a given day, or if I think I might need a real sound night's sleep, I might take a small (2–3 mg) "quality" melatonin pill thirty minutes before my intended sleep start.

I don't mind this little mellowing ritual, as natural melatonin is within us (just like cholesterol production). I take melatonin as needed, not as a nightly habit. No, I'm not fooled by the "natural equals safe" salesmanship we often see and hear in our screened digital lives. Be skeptical, too. Next, let's think about getting around.

WHAT IS MY TOP TRAVEL HACK FOR YOU?

Avoid time-zone tiredness by being as rested as possible *before* you start your trip. Yes, world travelers may want or need prescription sleeping aids so that jet lag doesn't turn them into zombies. If so, I merely ask them and you to think about possible side effects of sleep aids. Please consider natural ways to get sleep for your time at thirty-two thousand feet, and when you land in a different time zone.

Our circadian rhythms normally elevate our melatonin level after noon. Hence, midafternoon slumps of energy and temporary drowsiness may happen at about 3:00 p.m. for your normal, local time. Grab twenty winks or a *nappucino*. Then get back to your great, refreshed GenX day and night, whatever your time zone. How about noble grapes?

IS RED WINE MIGHTY FINE?

Yes, and no. Yes, to (*probably*) improve your heart health. And, no for sipping wine or spirits as sleep aids. Despite its documented antioxidant and mellowing aspects, wine may cause you *predawn* wakeups.

- Moderate your dinnertime and nightcap drinking of beer, spirits, or wine.

Redux: nightcaps may help you get to sleep, yet they generally cause you to stir and lose your deep sleep later.

In no way would I encourage you to start drinking for a personal sleep experiment. Live and learn as you see fit. Please try to form habits that help you gain those seven or more blissful hours on most nights! Let's consider what I call a sleep food as another X factor.

ONIONS AND CUPID?

Onions don't seem to promote my sleep in a big way, though some studies suggest the contrary for others. You might try them as natural sleep aid (if you're sleeping alone, or perhaps if your sleep partner shares 'em).

I try to eat my evening meals early enough to have a happy gut by pillow time. And my meals are not too spicy, being mindful of Satchel Paige's counsel about moderation. Aphro-whats?

What about foods and spices that are labeled or touted as "natural" aphrodisiacs? Yes, I say, try 'em. Why? Either as placebos or actual blood flow boosts, Aphrodite's natural foods and spices may help you get it on, or *Marvin Gaye* it, as they say. Then, better sleep may follow. Oxytocin and prolactin rise with a big or little *O*, while cortisol dreamily drops.

Please check what the credible Sleep Foundation has to say about intimate feeling, hormone releases and superior sleep. Sexercise and restorative sleep *do* correlate! Back to Aphrodite ... Eat her offerings to enjoy their taste and whatever consequences they *may* enable.

Here are some possible aphrodisiacs that you might consider. As always, be mindful of interactions if you take prescription drugs. And be mindful that what works for another GenX may not work for you.

- ✓ Zinc-rich oysters that you read about earlier
- ✓ Ginseng
- ✓ Dark chocolate
- ✓ Pistachios
- ✓ Maca
- ✓ Chili peppers.

Make sleep foods a great part of your restful sleep kit. For emphases, let's re-examine what excessive volume, intensity, and the tempo of strength training can have on your sleep.

OVERTRAINING EQUALS UNDER SLEEPING

Would you agree that sleep and exercise practices are integrated? Check out this web blog from the National Federations of Professional Trainers.[100] See www.nfpt.com/blog/integrating-slee p-exercise-mutual-improvements.

I *never* heard an Olympic champion say that the real key to his or her gold medal was sleep *deprivation*. But I did read that the amazing Edwin Moses banked ten hours of sleep daily for his tip-top athletic performances. His 122-straight victories (no, 122 is *not* a typo) in grueling 400-meter hurdle events is amazing. I don't think I've ever slept ten hours straight as an adult. And I'm certainly not invincible, as Moses was for nine years of elite competition. Just sayin' that *proper sleep matters* in greatness.

Overtraining impacts one's periodic rest and restoration as an awful after. *Too much* exertion can truly make you or me irritable, prone to illness or injury, inflamed, less interested in sexercising, and sleep deficient. I have been there and done that, and *that* is *not* at all wonderful.

Achieving your personal best requires a goodly mix of volume, intensity, and tempo that can put you *close to an edge* of overtraining. You may have a spouse or sleep partner whose own serotonin is also lowered by your fitful attempts to sleep with you when you are overtrained. Listen to your mind and body and try not to mess with your partner's serotonin. Check?

Your sleep is very much an active—not passive—process of great value. You and I can count those valuable ways at http://sleep.org. Check this resourceful website, please.

Simple things, such as sleeping like a baby, can be hard. Yet, managing stress (or distress) and gaining restorative sleep will help you optimize both your health span and lifespan. Onward, half a league onward with your sleepy capstone efforts. Enjoy your restful ROI. Those restorative ZZZs are a wonderful way to invest one-third of your life. Those ZZZs will sustain your strong GenX performances.

Do *not* forget that Swiss army knife of sleep. Restorative sleep *is* your physical banking capstone. In closing for this uber-significant X factor, think about this nourishing English literature course:

"Sleep, great nature's second course, chief nourisher in life's feast" (MacBeth, Act II, Scene II).

Would the Bard lie? Get on course to take *full* advantage of your "chief nourisher" and to keep motion as very good medicine.

SUBCHAPTER 4—MAKE MOBILITY MATTER

As a perpetual remembrance of September 11, 2001 events, it is useful to gauge mobility of "first responders" who devotedly help others.

Mobility matters greatly for first responders
who "live that they bear the strain."

Hustling a firehose up a stairwell in full firefighter gear is a mobility strain, I assure you. Rucking an eighty-pound pack in hot battle conditions is another strain.

Question: What mobility moves matter most for the tactical fitness of soldiers, marines, firefighters, and police officers?

Answer: First responders are very concerned with key moves for injury prevention and longevity of service.

So, *mobility moves that prevent injury* and help you keep on keepin' on matter most.

Our real-life action heroes must move through full ranges of tactical motion (ROM) when carrying their personal protective equipment (PPE) or when carrying someone in a firefighter's carry. In ways like those first responders and military folks, *you need mobility* to cope with unnatural or compromised positions, with or without additional weight carried. Please highlight this operational definition:

- **Mobility** is the functional movement of one or more of your skeletal joints, plus connective tissue, fascia, and muscles through a ROM.

Note that mobility is similar to, yet different from stretching or flexibility efforts which lengthen your muscles, fascia, and connective tissues. Here is a WIFM answer for your capable motion:

✓ Mobility can help you overcome joint restrictions, limited ROM, neural dysfunction, and even motor control problems.

Yes, there are some physical conditions that merit tailored programs for proper mobility. For example, joint hypermobility syndrome (JHS) is a rare condition for some people that requires tailored and interactive programming so that they can safely achieve and defend their ROM.

Dr. Kelly Starrett, founder of (TRS) The Ready State™,[101] or other fitness professionals, can coach you to correct any functional mobility restrictions you may face. One of Starrett's TRS blogs addresses aches and pains at the age of fifty or later. It merits this flexing consideration.

FLEX ALERT #28:

"It's not the high mileage running that … has you limping around each time you rise from your chair, or the military presses that caused your arm to ache each time you reach for something overhead. It's the *progressively sedentary* and less physically demanding lifestyles we adopted that have put us in this … Movement Poverty Predicament."[102]

I wish there was a simpler phrase than movement poverty predicament, yet a $10 Million GenX certainly does not want poverty!

Ouch. Don't fall into a sedentary and less-demanding *predicament* like this! Those sedentary comments of Starrett may fit in decent or good GenX folks. Conversely, great GenX folks avoid movement poverty predicaments for health span—correct?

Mobilize yourself with knowledge and proper movement to oil up your tinman or tin woman, please. Remember to get in the arena and use your full mobility as a tangible X factor.

I next cite a credible triad of mobility strengths from Aleks Salkin, a fitness professional known as "the Hebrew Hammer."[103]

- The ability to move odd objects through free space (this is resistance effort).
- The ability to move your body through free space (this is bodyweight effort).
- The ability to move your body the way it was originally *designed* to move (this is what the Hammer calls original strength.)

This third consideration, original strength (or OS), is *not* a software operating system. Rather, it is your primal movement and mobility as a mammal. OS is your wired capacity to move things that stand in your way.

Salkin offers six movements in his OS protocol that you should consider:

1. Breathing.
2. Neck nods.
3. Rolling.
4. Rocking.
5. Crawling.
6. Standing cross crawl.

Let's check on those two mobility crawls in numbers five and six of Salkin's protocol. Appreciate why and how these original strength (OS) crawls help with more advanced strength movements.

#5: A Bear crawl or "quadruped" plank is the starting position for a dynamic bear crawl. This crawl is a wonderful strength, stability, and stretch movement for your mobility. You can shift forward, backward, or sideways with opposite and alternating arm/leg crawling motions. I encourage you to regularly get down and crawl to emulate the mobility of a kid (or a brown bear.)

#6: A standing cross crawl sounds a bit confusing, yet this complex mobility move for OS is a warm-up for other yoga, stability, or strength moves.

- Stand with your feet spread slightly apart, perhaps at shoulder width. Raise your arms, with your shoulders relaxed. Inhale mindfully.
- Exhale as you bring your opposite elbow and knee toward each other in front of you. Tighten your abdominal core muscles with "belly button to spine" support for this front-to-back and twisting move.
- Inhale as you return to your starting position and one repetition is done.

This standing OS move with a strange-sounding name will become as easy for you as one, two, three.

OS Movements like numbers 1-4 were endorsed by a Ukrainian-born engineer named Moshe Feldenkrais. His Feldenkrais method (FM) requires a trained practitioner to guide a person through gentle *somatic* movements. (Somatic means "learning from within" and applies movement for movement's sake.) The FM goal is learning self-improved movements for ADL that stem from expanded perception and awareness of habits and tensions. If I piqued your interest in FM (which is *not* f#$%ing magic, by the way), please visit https://feldenkrais.com to learn more and possibly opt-in for newsletters.

I am researching how FM may help boost one's sense of self after a stroke, traumatic brain injury, or cerebral palsy. I want to help those sub-populations achieve better motion as medicine too.

You may have heard about Qigong as a free-form movement practice. This ancient technique is based on gentle movements with breathwork and is used by billions of people today. I leave details of FM and Qigong and other movement and learning techniques for your self- evaluation. I close this X Factor subchapter with your mobility wrap:

With your increased mobility and full ROM, *your weightlifting form will improve for both safety and performance.*

As you train with proper form and skeletal positioning, you get stronger and safer for ADLs. Just think of doing a pistol squat like a pro or show your grandkids that you can do a sit-to-rise move just like they can.

Do you agree that mobility matters for you as a strong GenX? Great. Now, on to select aids for your journey in your next subchapter.

SUBCHAPTER 5—FITNESS DEVICES AND APPLIANCES

As a prelude to your cursory look at "fitness" appliances and devices, please take this to heart: they *cannot* do the work for you.

Right, GenX is comfortable with technology advances in general, and "smart" mobile appliances or applications in particular. So, celebrate some smart applications that can aid you on your strong-to-save journey. However, to be repetitive, repetitive—you are the one who does the work, not your appliance or Elon Musk's new robot. Hmmm, are these devices pricey?

Maybe yes, maybe no. *Sticker shock* may result if you choose to invest in high-end, high-tech devices or appliances as your training aids. Become a savvy buyer in inflationary times. It is up to you whether to invest or not. And if you do invest, how high a price point is still right for you? I suggest that you settle on the functions and features you need in your appliance first. Then shop smartly for a price point that works for you. You do *not* have to make expensive purchases. Jack LaLanne never did. Nor Leonides or Braveheart. *What are you looking for?*

We know that computing devices calculate, communicate, and bookkeep. Well, you are likely looking for a device to accurately measure and report your heart rates, motions, or steps, and bookkeeps your nightly sleep results. More bells and whistles can certainly be purchased in America's land of plenty. You are the best judge of your needs or a wants in a fitness aid, rather than a Madison Avenue "mad man."

Buyer beware is a fitting platitude that may have a "ring" to it.

PRESENTED FOR MERIT:

I offer my personal experiences as testimonials for the benefits of some fitness devices.

My Oura™ ring used my body temperature, heart rate, heart rate variability, and respiration trends to suggest I wasn't right in the fall of 2022. Soon after, a painful, blistering shingles rash broke out on my torso. Those ring sensors were great scouts for my emergent shingles symptoms.

Likewise for my lone bout with a COVID-19 variant that was an unwanted souvenir from our summer 2023 vacation. My Oura Ring pegged high temperature, irregular breathing, higher heart rate, lower heart rate variability, plus poorer sleep quality many hours *before* I popped positive with a COVID-19 home test kit.

In addition, ladies in GenX who have not yet entered menopause may find that devices like an Oura ™ are quite good at predicting their monthly cycles.

Many folks now wear Fitness watches. I could name a long list of options for such devices. Or I can share with you what I opt to use. I wear a Fitbit™ Versa 3 model for my "smart watch." I *don't* use all of its razzle dazzle functions like music, payments, or previewing emails or text messages. Yet, it is always a nice "attaboy" when I get that subjective up check for my 10,000 steps. Each to his or her own...

Again, a worthy device need not be expensive. Think of a drug store purchase "on sale" or a credible (ad-free) smart phone application for your pulse and blood oxygen sensing. It is a good idea to monitor your heart rate and oxygen absorption regularly, yes? Is such an app or device expensive? No. *Is Digital the answer?* Sometimes.

ALSO TRIED AND TRUE:

I appreciate, use, and recommend analog devices too. For example:

- A great GenX should acquire a dynamometer to regularly check grip strength. Grip strength is a fascinating biomarker for one's general constitution and for dying harder when SARS viruses wing around you.
- The best heart rate monitor is a chest strap, perhaps a Garmin device. Knowing your heart rate for exertion is very important.

I know from experience that my unique thumper with "low" heart rates, can cause erroneous heart rate measures by my Oura ring or Fitbit watch in my workouts. So, I strap on something that is accurate and telling when I need to know how hard I'm working!

- Likewise, procure a *spirometer* as a portable breathing device to exercise your pulmonary muscles. Remember those Norwegians and their impressive VO_2 maximums.

Now, get ready to take a deep, nasal cleansing breath.

SUBCHAPTER 6—BREATH

Never forget to breathe with focus and purpose when you're weightlifting or doing other exercises or activities. It is a very good practice to extend this focus to nearly all your daily and nightly endeavors.

"Most people think that they're breathing when they're doing strength training exercises, but they may be holding their breaths. It's important to inhale and exhale fully between each repetition. The key is to *avoid straining* when holding your breath. You may find it helpful to exhale during the more strenuous phase of the exercise and inhale during the less strenuous phase."[104]

ENJOY THAT AIR YOU BREATHE

I highly recommend *Breath,* a New York Times best-selling book by James Nestor about mindful breathing. I believe you will benefit from a review of a "new science of a lost art." Mindful breathing that is ingrained in your exercise and ADLs is a key element of being "in the zone." Nestor's literary work is a wonderful read, and his journey to find the alternative to *bad breath,* so to speak, is a compelling trigger for you to also become a certified pulmonaut.

Lost art methods of breathing are vital for a strong GenX like you. Time-proven and athletically validated methods will help you breathe better, sleep better, perform better, and live longer. If you don't purchase Nestor's book, please visit his website[105] for video and audio tutorials to experience some or all of the eight breathing techniques listed below. There is no down side to getting calm in a flow zone – is there?

1. Diaphragm coordination
2. Alternate nostril breathing

Perform #2 for up to 5 minutes daily. This ancient technique is named Nadi Shodhanam Pranayama in Sanskrit. (I will call it alternate nostril breathing until my Sanskrit improves.)

3. Cardiac Coherent technique
   a. Inhale into your belly for five seconds.
   b. Exhale for another five seconds.
   c. Work up to repeat for three to five minutes. Breathe naturally, as you usually do, just slower.

4. Buteyko Breathing – as documented by a Ukrainian doctor in 1950.

Use your <u>diaphragm</u> for full body breathing instead of shallow chest breathing. When you do, you avoid hyperventilation and overproduction of carbon dioxide (CO_2).

5. Tummo Technique – try an ancient Tibetan meditation technique to build your "inner fire."

6. Sudarshan kriya yoga – sometimes called SKY yoga breathing.

7. I use the US Navy SEAL box breathing method of 4-4-4-4 seconds to calm my heart rate and lower my blood pressure when stressed. Take 4 box cycles of in, hold, out, pause and you're done in ~ a minute. Well, done in 64 seconds for one round.

8. The well-known technique of four, seven, eight-second breathing cited by Dr. Andrew Weil is also worthy of your trials. Inhale for 4 seconds, hold your deep breath for 7 seconds, then complete one cycle by slowly exhaling for 8 seconds. What a wonderful way to invest in your flow zone with nineteen seconds of your time.

Join me as a breather of the lost art. Your nose knows if you retrain it. Your optimal strength *is* a matter of life and breath! Now, back to natural curing in your next segment.

SUBCHAPTER 7—NATURE AND INTEGRATIVE MEDICINES

You have heard an expression that it is *not* nice to fool Mother Nature.

I assert that Mother Nature and her products are *not* fooling, as their X factors can boost your second half of life. Let's begin with a well-known holistic or integrative medicine, homeopathy. I share this established treatment of disease and conditions from my limited, yet *positive* experiences.

Cutting to the chase, an informed GenX *may* find relief in non-prescription, non-allopathic ways with natural cures. That is, temporary or lasting relief may be gained from ancient practices used by billions of people. Yes, I italicized *may*.

Fact: America was well-versed in practices of natural medicine until World War I. Then, two American billionaires named Rockefeller and Carnegie championed "new " western medicine and actively pilloried traditional medicines.

This is a sad yet true story. "Big Oil and Big Money" were triggers for this unfortunate sea change in business models as your recommended study of "The Flexner Report to Congress, 1910" will clearly show. Incidentally, the monopolistic American Medical Association was created at this time. Hmmm.

It is *our time* to take best practices and healing modalities - from wherever they originated - to fortify and defend our physical banking investments. Billionaires and governments are *not* always right.

HOMEOPATHY

The term homeopathy originated from two Greek words, *homoeos* and *pathos*, which mean "similar" and "suffering or disease" respectively.

Samuel Hahnemann, a German physician who practiced "modern, Western, or allopathic" medicine, observed that chinchona bark (quinine) served as a natural cure for malaria. This fortuitous observation led to his founding of homeopathy practices in 1790.[106]

Where does homeopathy stand today in comparison to "western" healing efforts? Pardon, yet ponder these two lengthy quotes as answers:

"Homeopathy is used by just over 2 percent of the U.S. population ... Recent clinical trials highlight several areas in which *homeopathy may play a role* in improving public health, including infectious diseases, pain management, mental health, and cancer care."[107]

"Homeopathy users, particularly those who also report visiting homeopathic practitioners, find the use of these products helpful and that they tend to use a greater variety of complementary and integrative medicine (CIM) modalities than do users of supplements and other

CIMs. This is the first detailed report on the use of homeopathy in this country."[108]

Am I a CIM fan? Why, *yes*, I am. Will I consider a homeopathic treatment from a practitioner if and when I face an infectious disease or bodily pain? You betcha.

Doctor Hahnemann established three cardinal rules or laws for modern homeopathy. Quick citations are listed for each of these principles.

- **Law of Similia**: this rule is shorthand for "let like be treated by likes."[109] A case in point: I find it fascinating that poison ivy extract, called Rhus toxicodendron (Rhus Tox, or Rhus-T for short), is a homeopathic remedy for select symptoms *like* skin irritation, auto-immune pain, and some fevers.
- **Law of Simplex:** a patient is administered only one homeopathic remedy at a time. A practitioner is trained to prioritize and sequence single remedies in order. Bear in mind that a person taking prescription drugs from Western practices might be advised by the homeopathic practitioner to suspend that regimen to let homeopathy take its course without side effects, This special case is definitely one when a physician should be consulted. Above all, do no harm!
- **Law of Minimum Dose:** homeopathic treatments from natural sources are administered in *sub-physiological* doses. There is a fancy word, posology, which means an appropriate dosage of a remedy. Dr. Hahnemann and his many homeopathic successors have evolved very *minimal* doses to excite the body's vital force or energy.

Yes, this third rule has a hint of alchemy and elixir magic at first glance. Yet billions of people on our planet rely on such tiny dosages to prompt their energy centers to heal them or reduce symptoms naturally.

Of course, this minimal law generates *"highly diluted"* humor...

Example: The less I rely on homeopathic medicine, the better off I am. ...*I guess it works.*

As a student of my endeavor, I now consider traditional medicine to heal me or to reduce symptoms of a condition like fungal nail infections. Under the advice of a practitioner, my *guess* is that I may save money and get better without western prescriptions.

FULL DISCLOSURE

I am *not* a practitioner of *similias*. I include this information for your own evaluation of traditional and Western medicines. I want to aid your search for complements or alternatives to "western" medicines as CIM for both health care and sick care. Note that I intentionally segregate *sick care* and health care. I advocate natural lifestyles with minimal polypharmacy for healthcare. That is, to the extent possible until sickness dictates otherwise.

I tried a homeopathic remedy from a practitioner for joint pain and my chronic rower's elbow in recent years. I do not know how effective the homeopathic remedy, called Ruta Graveolens or Ruta was, as I was also undergoing physical therapy at that time. Yet my symptoms notably improved. For that end result I am thankful.

Most recently, I accepted the homeopathic recommendation of a certified practitioner for a carefully contrived sulfur potion to alleviate both my sinusitis and fungal athlete's foot. And yes, my symptoms were greatly reduced. Sure, this a tiny sample size and one must always be attuned to side effects. However,...

I want to avoid prescription drugs unless I need them for do-or-die sick care regimens. (Now, at age seventy in 2023, I am blessed that I take zero prescription drugs, while I still take stairsteps two at a time.) Traditional CIM *may* help me maintain this lifestyle without polypharmacy for many moons. Or it may not...

Here's a worldly view of homeopathy from the other side of

the Atlantic. I have a wonderful personal training client of French descent. She shared that her compatriots, plus Europeans in general, accept non-Western remedies more than Americans. *Arnica* (a genus in the sunflower family), is her homeopathic go-to remedy if diarrhea or inflamed muscles impact her ADLs.

I do like the holistic approach of homeopathy that advises a practitioner to make close observations of the entire symptoms of a patient, rather than the acute or localized symptom.

One note of caution: You may have a sensitivity or allergy to a plant-based or mineral medicine (in either homeopathic or allopathic approaches.) Please become knowledgeable and innovative as you consider "healing" plants or minerals.

Repeat after me: homeopathic remedies are not for amateurs and its stringent processes need to be followed for proper, effective use.

In my book, homeopathy was and is still worth pursuit for problems that I face on my strength journey. That may or may not be the case for you, and that is perfectly fine. It does not seem to be snake oil, although there is a homeopathic remedy that originates from viper venom—yup!

Note: I omitted some traditional practices like ancient Ayurvedic healings that comprise elements of nutrient, diet, exercise, and lifestyle. I have not experienced those approaches. Next ...

ESSENTIAL OILS FOR HEALING

By this point, you know that I appreciate old and new, analog and digital, eastern and western. You now grasp that I like natural approaches to boost your strong performance. You sense that I am open to alternatives for Western medicine and what I call expensive "sick care." Homeopathic essential oils (and herbs) have been used by our forebears across millennia to aid digestion and promote sleep, and to counter inflammation, discomfort, or pain. *Au naturel* oils appeal to me as "pain killers" do.

- **Capsaicin oil.** First, when eaten with moderation, peppers with capsaicin are good for your microbiome (gut). Next, if you haven't tried capsaicin as a topical oil, a cream, or liquid roll-on for soreness or pain, *you should* (in my opinion). For many folks like me, capsaicin on your skin beats taking a NSAID to counter delayed onset of muscle soreness or DOMS. *I used topical capsaicin to alleviate the "religious" symptoms of my shingles.* But be sure to keep the peppery treatment away from eyes or sensitive body parts!
- **Ginger oil.** Ginger is a fine anti-inflammatory root (or rhizome) for topical and diffused use. Its oils can be potent, so you want to follow directions for their proper dilution.
- **Peppermint oil and eucalyptus oil.** These two essential oils offer similar aromatic and anti-inflammatory properties. I am sure that some of you have other oils that you leverage, too. These oils can be pricey, so shop around for possible discounts on quality bottles.
- **Lavender oil.** As with soothing chamomile tea, diffused lavender oil is widely thought to be a soothing sleep enhancer. Some folks combine small melatonin doses with these oils for better sleep.

HERBS AND SPICES FOR HEALING

As for your other X factors, I am not writing *soup to oils to nuts* in an unabridged way. I summarize just the anti-inflammatory and disease-fighting herbs and spices of merit that I use. As a quick spicy example, I do ingest Boswellia or frankincense. Right, this is the biblically cited frankincense. My rationale is – why not check an

Indian ayurvedic remedy and a gift of the Magi to counter joint pain and inflammation?

I skip others, including one of the oldest medicinal plants that we know, aloe vera. Too much good stuff is out there to incorporate in these healing pages.

Great! If you are interested in natural healing, you will find those plants, herbs, spices, and oils that soothe and heal you.

- Make a note that about one-third of placebos do have clinically measured results.

Whether as placebo or as actual healing, my experiential approach is to give ancient and natural remedies a chance to help me, despite what John Rockefeller championed.

FLEX ALERT #29:

Three-fourths of the world's population relies on holistic and herbal medicine as a primary source of medical care. 3/4ths!

What about us Westerners in the other 1/4? Are there *adaptogens* (i.e., plants and mushrooms) that can help our bodies respond to stress too? *Yes.*

- **Herbal essences.** Chilis, cumin, parsley, cilantro, and basil are wonderful herbs that offer you vitamin and mineral micronutrients. I commend to you a fine resource titled *Best Herbs for Healing* by Robert McCaleb that ranks and rates plants used in fresh, dried, or extracted form to promote, maintain, or restore health.

  McCaleb makes me re-think some assumptions about Western medicine: "In our haste to embrace 'scientific' medicine, we quickly forgot the contributions nature makes to medicine." *Don't you forget Mother Nature.*

I pay into our nation's health care system (Medicare.) And today I stand to benefit from Medicare's sick-care coverage as needed. Please don't get me wrong. I am a cheerleader for great western medicine men and women, as I may be their sick-care patient one day, but not yet ... What else may be nice?

- **Spice is nice.** Cinnamon to curcumin, clove to cardamom, and Himalayan salt to black pepper are selected spices that I advocate for health span and lifespan. Some spices like trusted black pepper enhance the absorption of other micronutrients in your body. Many help you keep your taste buds excited with sweet and umami senses. You may find that you can use less sugar, oil, and salt in your home-cooking when spices are added.

  Cinnamon is also a fine topper for coffee and hot chocolate. What's *not* to love about a tasty anti-inflammatory topper? And what is not to love about *nature's contributions* that just might transform you?

SUBCHAPTER 8—XFORMERS

The epitaph on Jack LaLanne's headstone says it all:

It's better to wear out than rust out.

Did you know that Mrs. LaLanne is still active at age 97 as I write Strong to Save?

Even *little* quantities of exercise can generate major positive effects, *despite* bodily wear and tear. Along with the LaLannes, I underscore the interrelationship of "wearing" exercise and health to fight dementia-related diseases (DRD) and offer a proven fighter's recipe.

Consider one DRD, namely Alzheimer's disease (AD).
Is there a secret sauce of exercise to counter DRD
and AD? Here it is: "Frequent exercise for 6–8 weeks
lessens the risk of dementia development."[109]

This follow-on should sound familiar to you.

"Exercise intervention to prevent dementia requires *appropriate exercise patterns based on individual* health and physical condition, as well as adhering to the principles of progressive load, overload, and specificity of exercise training."[110]

Amen. These are appealing "*lessens,*" aren't they?

✓ Your just-right exercise also serves as an effective intervention for anxiety and some other depression disorders. It is tragic that depression affects healthspans of so many in Gen X – perhaps 5 %. That percentage equates to millions of sufferers! And sadly, women are diagnosed more often than men.

My Rx: Shift from polypharmacy to poly-workouts. Or at least exercise in individualized programs as a credible and viable complement to DRD prescriptions.

One more soapbox speech of mine follows:

Many in GenX take multiple prescription drugs each and every day. Some are undoubtedly needed. Perhaps some prescriptions are unnecessary. Please beware of escalating drug costs, known and unknown side effects, and unintended consequences. I now ask a rhetorical query.

Is there a potential alternative or adjunct to polypharmacy for DRD and other brain-body conditions?

Naturally:

✓ Your brain can favorably change; just look up *neuroplasticity* on Doctor Google. [111]

Yes, our brains are malleable and can adapt to life's experiences with exercise that "feeds your head," as Grace Slick sang.

Yes, your brain can favorably adapt, even after bad things happen to good people. Think of cognitive behavior therapies. Imagine the benefits of pet therapy. We all need friends, and sometimes a furry friend is just the right prescription! Shifting from DRDs, lets next build on this "feed your head" theme.

Consider that legendary commencement speech by Navy Admiral William McRaven to University of Texas students and friends:[112]

MAKE YOUR BED

Grasp how you bring significant changes to your life through simple, early actions. McRaven later authored a successful book about such simple rituals or habits to make your day successful almost every day. *Make your bed* before you face a day's known and unknown challenges. Get yourself focused and pointed toward your goal line, as I do, with this **MORNINGS** mnemonic:

> **M**—Make your bed. Get that early success.

> **O**—Observe your resting heart rate, heart rate variability (if you have a fitness device) stress level, and urine clarity (seriously.) And observe your mindful breathing as you do your Good Morning salutation stretch.

> **R**—Reflect, ponder yesterday's accomplishments and today's *smart* objective to meet or exceed. And think just a minute about today's action plan.

N—Nutrients. Macros, micronutrients, and vital water. If you aren't intermittently fasting, eat the colors of the rainbow, and get plenty of H_2O.

I—Invigorate with a quick-yet-mindful yoga sun salutation series and take a hot-and-cold shower to help your "forgotten" lymphatic system function better. And hum while you're showering to activate your vital *vagus* nerve. Shake out those cobwebs. Do a Tony Robbins warm-up or a Monkey Paw stretch series.

N—Note one network connection or resource to help you on your strength journey. Make a social outreach by an eNote or text message to that noted connection.

G—Gratitude. Your cortisol level is harnessed when you are in a thankful, glass-is-half-full mindset. Mad-ons about things you cannot control in this zany world do not aid your *cause cele'bre*. Be grateful for lemons that make lemonade.

S—Signs. Jot a Post-It™ note as a reinforcing sign or marker. Here's one or my favorite signs I posted in my work area:

"Am I going to ride the waves or ignore them today?"

Mornings can be deal-makers for your cornerstone strengths and physical banking. Optimize your rise and shine times with this MORNINGS mnemonic checklist or implement one of your own design. It is harder to be anxious or depressed when you have successful morning habits. Check!

FLEX ALERT #30:

Checklists matter. Use checklists to journal your sthenic achievements and to note those accolades you collect for your changing physique and performance. Yes, you can!

Further, as Admiral McRaven shared, you must banish doubt, and take prudent risks to advance your GenX physical bank and your longer life. Banish the FUD – fear, uncertainty, and doubt. Positive, unwavering attitude is also an X Factor to reckon with.

As your new day progresses, whether you are a morning lark, night hawk, or third bird by nature, exit your comfort zone and explore your **Mission: I'm Possible.** Don't forget what Eleanor Roosevelt advised: "Do one thing every day that scares you."

Now, circle back to your MBA and mind-muscle connections (as discussed in chapter 6.) Think of your proven ways to "get into the flow, or zone." Consider how to keep your mind engaged and nimble. Know how to adapt and thrive 'til your final gun sounds. Embrace three malleable factors in Table 8.2 to improve your MBA and put forth strong performances in your many sthenic years to come:

Challenge and Novelty	Tackle something new and not too easy to learn.
Intention	Celebrate your feeling of reward for tackling a new, nontrivial task. ✓ Get dressed with your eyes closed. ✓ Brush your teeth with your less-dominant hand. ✓ Take different walking, biking, or driving routes. ✓ Frequent different stores when you shop. Mix it up …
Repetition and Intensity	One-and-done is *not* enough. Shorter bouts of intense repetition are usually needed to create new brain connections.

Table 8.2: Factors for Mission: I'm Possible

Immersive exercises—those that make you adapt and think—powerfully align your body, muscles, and mind. So, go ahead and mix up your strength workouts too. Feed your head and polish up that MBA.

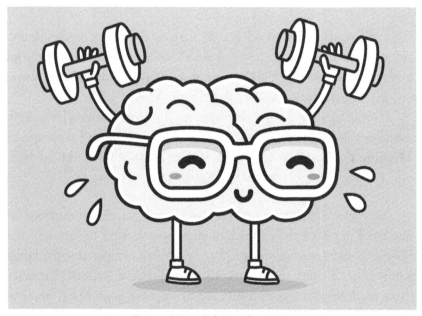

Figure 8.3: Polish Up That MBA

Hard work, even in small chunks, can be key to your successful second-half achievements. Check off these simple-yet-hard action steps to become strong to save:

- Commit to SMART objectives (*specific, measurable, achievable, realistic,* and *time-bound*).
  Don't set broad goals like "I want to be strong" or "I want to look good in a mirror." Codify *specific* and *attainable* objectives to help you stay motivated and to provide steppingstones of success.

- Be a lifelong learner as a student of your endeavor.
  Adopt an open mind to discover and try new things. Don't shy away from difficulty or challenge, as Eleanor Roosevelt advised.

- Make vital connections.
  Build strong professional ties to keep current with developments. I never got dumber by listening and emulating my role models' actions.

- Stay the course.
  Strength success just doesn't come suddenly. *Think about how long it took a skinny Austrian kid named Arnold to get shredded as the Terminator.*
  Don't get bogged down by your failures. Learn from those missteps or setbacks and celebrate your successes as Jack LaLanne did well into his nineties.

LIVE LONGER AND DIE HARDER AS AN XERCIST.

Yes, I conjured up that term *Xercist*. It wasn't Stan Lee's cunning.

Gain and maintain your *sthenic* functional strength from habitual motion, mobility, and moving heavy things. Live up to a book dedication for *You, Staying Young* by Dr. Mehmet Oz, and Dr. Michael Roizen.[113] Yes, one coauthor is *"that"* Doctor Oz.

"To all who desire a longer life so that they can serve more."

Serving more is a fine mantra of a great GenX who is strong to save. That sounds to me like YOU. As a great GenX, you control your attitude, from morning to night, in work and play. Yes, it is you who controls your work ethic.

Think of what you've read thus far in this fit map for health span and lifespan gains. Manifest its lessons, tips, and hacks to improve both your health span and lifespan, please.

Can you down age? I argue that you can gain a decade of vital years by staying strong, eating clean, and chasing Morpheus. Yea verily. Tangible X factors help you build and maintain your muscle manifesto.

Another key in your demonstrated manifesto is to have the courage, persistence, and grit to try again after you miss a mark. *If you are waiting for me to offer wisdom from the great John Wooden, it is written in your final chapter...*

Remember Dara Torres's opening quote in *Strong to Save*.

> Remember that positive Jedi challenge to do, not to try.

And remember TINA. <u>T</u>here <u>is</u> <u>n</u>o <u>a</u>lternative for strength training. Well, there is if you consciously choose to die earlier and easier!

It is just about time to end with new beginnings. Turn your page.

Nunc Coepi

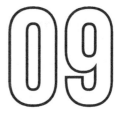

"Success is the sum of small efforts, repeated day in and day out."

—Robert Collier, author

We'll get to success and repetition in a moment. But first, do you wonder what *Nunc Coepi* means?

I did. This Latin phrase means "now I begin." Why do I devote your closing chapter of *Strong to Save* to what ancient Romans once uttered at their starting lines?

Because progress, or moving down the field, starts again with every play and habitual action. Because repetition of good habits, however small will lead to success as Admiral McRaven told Texas Longhorn graduates.

I could cite the relevant backings of stoics, who knew the merits of working body and mind, time and again. Or I could cite the case of another great GenX from America's biggest sport, professional football. Let me begin with that big time, great GenX.

A professional's professional, one Philip Rivers, the longtime San Diego Chargers quarterback is that great GenX. He is a shoo-in to wear the coveted yellow blazer of a National Football League Hall of Fame inductee.

Philip Rivers set thirty club records with San Diego, and then the Los Angeles Chargers. Not too shabby. He led the Indianapolis Colts to the league playoffs in his final campaign.

✓ Make consistency another X factor for your success.

Learn from his new beginnings as a fellow GenX and apply them to your own *Strong to Save* manifesto.

An eighteenth-century philosopher and scholar, Father Bruna Lanteri, wrote what became Philip Rivers' mantra,

"If I should fall ... a thousand times ... I will say immediately, *Nunc Coepi*."[114]

No matter what transpired, whether his best effort was a success or a flop, Philip Rivers had the resilience and focus to resolve, reboot, and begin again. He often wore his *Nunc Coepi* ballcap in public to stoically stress the importance of new beginnings.

Nunc Coepi still governs Philip Rivers' approach as he shifts away from the game he played so well for so long. Perseverance like his can and should be a personal strength habit for you as a strong GenX.

BEGIN ANEW

You're not alone when you strive to follow big footsteps of a resilient Philip Rivers or another GenX role model. Did you per chance follow NFL quarterback Tom Brady as another GenX who may just be the GOAT (or the greatest of all time) in his profession?

- How about Venus Williams, you ask?
- Or another court legend, Roger Federer?
- Or gymnast Mary Lou Retton who amazed us all with her injured vault in the LA '84 Olympics?
- Plus, you already know my admiration for Dara Torres, Dwayne Johnson, and Paralympian Todd Vogt as other GenX greats.

You don't need to be a professional to shine brightly for the next fifty years or so. However, you do *not* want to be an amateur, either, in your critical matter of fitness.

Could Socrates be wrong? I think not. Get a grip on his timeless thought from twenty-five centuries ago:

*"It is a shame to grow old without seeing the beauty
and strength of which you are capable."*

Your second-half success for both beauty and strength rests in your hands and mind. Do not suffer shame. Capably move stuff that stands in your way. Be strong to help others in our somewhat crazy world.

Samuel Clemens, aka Mark Twain, is another GOAT in my book as America's greatest author. With knowledge and humor, Twain advised:

"the secret of getting ahead is getting started."

I don't like to keep secrets, so I share my challenge to help you get started: *Begin anew*. Do the heavy work. Make it fun. Live longer and live better.

FLEX ALERT #31:

About 80 percent of New Year's resolutions become *unresolved* by each Valentine's Day. So, I ask two questions:

a. What caused that 80 percent of well-intentioned goal setters to miss the mark?
b. What goes right with those *other* 20 percent of sticky resolutions past each Valentine's Day?

Take a power ten, as we say in rowing. *Start right and you just might stay right on!*

These power 10 plus 1 guidelines *resolve* your "start right" plans and actions at any time of year, *and* in any of your encore years to come:

1. Choose specific micro goals. Set measurable and specific targets to hit. Re-calibrate your new targets and progress.

2. Chase the right stuff. Make resolutions of profound importance to *you*, like Philip Rivers did and does.

3. Journal. Regularly record both your successes and challenges in strength training and in your ADLs. Assess, adapt, achieve!

4. Give yourself a little slack. Practice patience and forgiveness through your inevitable *downs and ups* of life. Accept imperfections in others and in yourself. Reaffirm that you are on the right path to stay strong to save. Teddy Roosevelt and others cut you that slack; if you are in the arena, right? Efforts can generate errors. Learn from 'em and *Nunc Coepi*.

    If you miss a performance mark, show others your mojo and grit to get back in the arena to get it done.

5. Make the time. To be repetitive, *repetitive*, you must do the work you codified in your muscle manifesto. Remember that strength workouts can be very time-effective and efficient. Yet they do demand investment banking. Do not make excuses.

6. Skip solo routines. After all, the Lone Ranger relied on Tonto to ride again. Build your strong network with folks you trust to plan and execute your healthy meals, exercise, sleep, or new activities.

7. Commit fixed and discretionary resources. Yes, a kettlebell costs about $1.50 per pound, yet it lasts forever or nearly so. Focus on those important enablers to keep you strong, even if you forego old pleasures. Immerse yourself in work that can be fun and rewarding. Make Socrates's ghost happy as you maintain a strong body and nimble mind in your $10 Million portfolio.

8. Don't lose sight of why you set your resolution in the first place. Take a few deep breaths, defog your mind, celebrate your MBA, and rekindle your resolve each day. Dare I repeat, *Nunc Coepi?*

9. Reward yourself for achievements. Celebrate your victories on a regular basis. For examples:

     "Woot! I just carried my total bodyweight for a thirty-yard farmer's walk. I am functionally strong!"

     Or "I did my first Turkish Get-up with a heavy kettlebell."

     Or "I just did a pistol squat in great form."

     Or "I almost completed that one-minute pullup. I'll get that strength measure done in the next two weeks."

     Party on, then progress until you cannot.

10. Ask others to keep you accountable. Remember the Olympic gold network of New Zealand's Michael Brake that helped him *count and account* his physical banking efforts.

Find and leverage that workout buddy, professional trainer, coach, life partner, or whomever it may be help you count your bodily investments. And, you may remember an iconic basketball coach, John Wooden, who held even the free-spirited Bill Walton accountable. One of his many amazing comments about life and facing adversity is this:

"Failure to change might be fatal."

Who is that alter-ego of yours for true accountability and for being your change agent to avert failure? Here is your bonus:

+1. Mirror your new beginning. Is that man or woman in your mirror the one you know you can be? If not, take Dr. Oz's and Michael Jackson's counsel to make your world a better place.

Strong to Save will help you begin anew to:

- ✓ understand the WIFM of resistance training as medicine, very good medicine, to downage your health span and lifespan.
- ✓ be a good student to train your little mice to offset sarcopenia.
- ✓ lift, push, pull, twist, and carry bodyweight or resistance objects through full ranges of motion (ROM.)
- ✓ move stuff or move yourself in three body planes.
- ✓ look good and perform well by day and night, proving that Sexercise is good Gen X exercise.
- ✓ leverage your X Factors to be the best that you can be for another half-century of vibrant life.

As you close in on the last Period of Strong to Save, re-flex your mind and body one more time…

FINAL FLEX ALERT #32:

The word origin of *manifest*o is "obvious." If you see obvious merits in a personal manifesto as I do, please start your own muscle manifesto. Then journal your *obvious* investments on your strength journey.

Flag this final point, please:

Your journal doesn't need to be fancy.

It *plainly* and professionally holds you accountable for what it takes to win in your down-aged way of life. A manifesto will help you pursue and celebrate your impeccable strong performances for years to come. That manifesto clearly establishes your WIFM.

My own manifesto started with the declaration that I would overcome a "fuse my spine at forty-nine" malady. Two decades later, I'm staying well past forty and doing my darndest to stretch my vital health span years.

Are you ready to boldly state who you are and who you hope to become? Where are you now in your strength journey?

- What, if anything, is standing in your way?
- What investment of time, talent, and discretionary treasure are you willing to make?
- What will attaining your *strong-to-save* goal mean for your second half of life?

I cannot think of a better takeaway, as you wrap up your fit map, to make resisted motion your very good medicine than this:

The E.N.D. (The Energy Never Dies).

I extend my everlasting thanks to the Black-Eyed Peas for this E.N.D., this energetic closure.

Join other great GenX listeners and make tonight a good, good night.

Fuel your dreams.
Move what stands in your way.
Make motion your very good medicine.
Make your second half of life your "better half."
Die Harder and later. TINA.

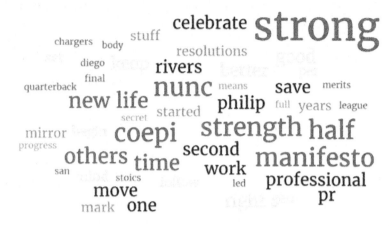

Figure 9.1: Die Harder and Later

Stay strong - well past forty.
—Dave Frost

Glossary of Abbreviations in Strong to Save

Introduction

PD. Parkinson's Disease.
Sthenic. Having a high or excessive level of strength and energy.
PRN. When necessary.
TINA. There is no alternative.

Chapter 1

Kinetic. Put something into motion.
PPST3. Practical programming for Strength Training.
TGU. Turkish get up.
NFPT. National Federation of Professional Trainers.
SSC. Stretch shortening cycle.
S.A.I.D. Specific adaptation to imposed demands.
D.E.E.P. Dynamic Endured Explosive Peak strengths.

Chapter 2

GOAT. Greatest of all time.
DOMS. Delayed onset of muscle soreness.
F.I.T.T. Four specific strength factors: frequency, intensity, time, and type.
SLDL. Single Leg Dead Lift.
NSCA. National Strength and Conditioning Association
1RM. One Repetition Maximum.
HP or hp. Horsepower.
EPOC. Excess Postexercise Oxygen Consumption.
Kcal. A dietary calorie.

WIFM. What's in it for me?

Pvt. Tim Hill. Nine essential amino acids.

ASCVD. Atherosclerosis/Cardiovascular disease.

BMI. Body-mass index or indicator.

MetS. Metabolic syndrome.

NAFLD. Nonalcoholic fatty liver disease.

CVD. Cardiovascular disease.

NFL. National Football League.

LEAN. Acronym for

    L—lighten.

    E—enhance.

    A—activate.

    N—nurture.

ADL. Activities of daily life.

StR. Sit to Rise longevity check.

Chapter 3

CNS. Central nervous system.

PNS. Peripheral nervous system.

MD. Doctor or medicine.

NTNU CERG. The Norway University of Science and Technology/Cardiac Exercise Research Group.

1RM. One repetition maximum.

ROS. Reactive oxygen species, aka oxidative free radicals.

TLF. Testosterone-limiting factor.

BPA. Bisphenol A (BPA)—a industrial chemical that may be harmful.

NMD. Neuromuscular disorder.

PD. Parkinson's disease.

MS. Multiple sclerosis.

MD. Muscular dystrophy.

ROM. Range of motion.

Chapter 4

ATP. Adenosine triphosphate.
psi or PSI. Pounds per square inch (pressure).
MBA. Mind-body alignment.
TVA. Transverse abdominus.
IO. Internal oblique.
TFL. Tensor fascia latae.
PNS. Peripheral nervous system.
TLFs. Testosterone-limiting factors.
Stat. Right now.
ATP. Adenosine triphosphate.
DBS. Dormant butt syndrome.
WOD. Workout of the day (CrossFit™).
PR. Personal record/Personal best.
CRAAP-tested. Current, relevant, authoritative, accurate, and published.
H&S. Hypertrophy and strength.
LPHC. Lumbo pelvic hip complex.
GT. Gluteus medius tendinopathy.
DBS. Dormant butt syndrome.
SI. Sacroiliac joint.
DVT. Deep-vein thrombosis.
Gmax. Gluteus maximus.
CTA. Call to action.
PED. Performance enhancing drug.

Chapter 6

HODL. Hold on for dear life.
MBA. Mind-body alignment.
PA. Physical activity.
TuT. Time under tension.

Chapter 7

VITA workout. Volume, intensity, tempo, adapt/alter.
Vitamin P. Natural micronutrients that are plant-based.
UV. Ultra-violet.
HRV. Heart rate variability.
ECGC. A healthy tea catechin.
LDL. Low-density lipoprotein.
HIIT. High-intensity interval training.
NO. Nitric oxide.
NSAID. Nonsteroidal anti-inflammatory drug.
CBD. Nonhallucinogenic cannabidiol.
THC. Psychoactive compound of cannabis.
PTSD. Post-traumatic stress disorder.
AREDS 2. Age-related eye disease studies—eye vitamins.
MDR. Minimum daily requirement.
MCTQ. Munich chronotype questionnaire.
IFE. Intermittent fasting for exercise.
EPOC. Excess postexercise oxygen consumption.
CPAP. Continuous positive airway pressure.
OSA. Obstructive sleep apnea.

Chapter 8

ROM. Ranges of tactical motion.
PPE. Personal protective equipment.
OS. Original strength.
CIM. Complementary and *integrative medicine*.
DRD. Dementia-related diseases.
AD. Alzheimer's disease.
FM. Feldenkrais method.

Chapter 9

GOAT. Greatest of all time.

Endnotes

Chapter 1

1 https://www.masterclass.com/articles/single-leg-deadlift-guide.
2 Daniel J. Levitin, *Successful Aging* (New York: Penguin Random House, 2020), 287.

Chapter 2

3 P. Mergenthaler, U. Lindauer, G. A. Dienel, A. Meisel. "Sugar for the Brain: The role of Glucose in Physiological and Pathological Brain Function," *Trends Neuroscience* 2013 36, no. 10 (October 2013):587–97. doi: 10.1016/j.tins.2013.07.001.
4 https://www.nationalgeographic.com/history/article/ 141029-amazo ns-scthians-hunger-games-herodotus-ice-princess-tattoo-cannabis for nonmythical Amazon women.
5 https://www.afar.org/what-is-geroscience
6 https://peterattiamd.com/mikejoyner
7 S.Hody, et al., Eccentric Muscle Contractions: Risks and Benefits. Front Physiol.2019 May 3,10: 536.doi: 10.3389/ fphys.2019.00536. PMID:31130877;PMCID:PMC6510035.
8 Jette M, Sidney K, Blumchen,G. Metabolic equivalents (METS) in exercise testing, exercise prescription, and evaluation of functional capacity. Clin Cardiol. 1990 Aug;13(8):555–65.doi:10.1002/clc.4960130809.PMID: 2204507.
9 American College of Sports Medicine. *ACSM's Guidelines for Exercise Testing and Prescription.* New York: Lippincott Williams & Wilkins, 2013.
10 https://www.verywellfit.com/f-i-t-t-principle-what-you-need-for -great-workouts-1231593
11 https://www.bionity.com/en/encyclopedia/ somatotype.html
12 https://a-z-animals.com/blog/discover-the-monomers-and-polymers-of-protein-plus-tips-for-remembering-them/
13 https://www.talkingaboutmenshealth.com/waist-to-hip-ratio-vs-bmi-wh y-you-might-discount-one-mass-measurement/

14 WHO. (2008). *Waist circumference and waist–hip ratio: report of a WHO expert consultation.* Geneva: World Health Org. http://apps.who.int/iris/bitstream/ handle/ 10665/44583/9789241501491_eng.pdf;jsessionid=E1530BB1E964 D66EC4AB4DE9E41147DC?sequence=1

15 Watson, S. (2021). Waist-to-Hip Ratio: Chart, Ways to Calculate, and More. https://www.healthline.com/health/ waist-to-hip-ratio

16 https://www.hopkinsmedicine.org/health/conditions-and-diseases/ adrenal-glands

17 Jarred Moon, "Murphy's Law, Fitness Edition: Can you be better?"https:// www.endofthreefitness.com/murphys-law-fitness-edition-can-you-be-better/

18 Rosenberg I. Summary comments: epidemiological and methodological problems in determining nutritional status of older persons. *Am J Clin Nutr.* 1989;50:1231–3.

19 Eske, J. (2021). Muscle atrophy: Causes, symptoms, and treatments. https://www.medicalnewstoday.com/articles/ 325316

20 Metzl, J., & Barrow, K. (2021). The 9-Minute Strength Workout. https:// www.nytimes.com/guides/well/strength-training-plyometrics

Chapter 3

21 https://psychology.fandom.com/wiki/Urinary_incontinence

22 C.P. Ko, Neuromuscular system, International Encyclopedia Of the Social & Behavioral Sciences, Pergamon, 2001.

23 Cynthia Cross, "Strengthen Your Nervous System the Natural Way: 10 Tips." https://www.top10homeremedies.com/how-to/how-to-strengthen-your-nervous-system.html

24 www.eparmedx.com. (2019). *The Physical Activity Readiness Questionnaire for Everyone* (Ebook). http://eparmedx.com/wp-content/uploads/2013/03/ FINAL-FILLABLE-ParQ-Plus-Jan-2019.pdf

25 https://www.worldfitnesslevel.org/#/

26 Cherry, K. (2020). What to Know About Nature vs. Nurture. https://www. verywellmind.com/what-is-nature-versus-nurture-2795392

27 Maine, M., & Kelly, J. *The Body Myth.* Hoboken, N.J.: John Wiley & Sons, 2005.

28 https://www.nfpt.com/blog/how-to-stimulate-cellular-renewal

29 Nomikos, N., Nikolaidis, P., Sousa, C., Papalois, A., Rosemann, T., & Knechtle, B. (2018). Exercise, Telomeres, and Cancer: "The Exercise-Telomere Hypothesis". *Frontiers In Physiology, 9.* doi: 10.3389/fphys.2018.01798

30 Macmillan, A. (2021). Exercise Makes You Younger at the Cellular Level. https://time.com/4776345/exercise-aging-telomeres/

31 https://www.cdc.gov/nutrition/micronutrient-malnutrition/micronu trients/index.html

32 https://www.parkinson.org/Understanding-Parkinsons/Causes/ Environmental-Factors

33 https://www.nhs.uk/conditions/multiple-sclerosis/

Chapter 4

34 https://www.britannica.com/science/skeletal-muscle

35 Ivanenko, Yury, and Victor S Gurfinkel. "Human Postural Control." Frontiers in neuroscience vol. 12 171. 20 March. 2018, doi:10.3389/ fnins.2018.00171.

36 Knight K. (2016). Muscle revisited. *J. Exp. Biol.* 219, 129– 133. 10.1242/ jeb.136226

37 http://www.jokes4us.com/sportsjokes/weightliftin gjokes.html

38 http://www.jokes4us.com/sportsjokes/weightliftin gjokes.html

39 Carpenter, Hayden. How to Progress into a Pistol Squat. *Outside.* https://www.outsideonline.com/health/training-performance/ how-do-pistol-squat/

40 M, S. (2021). Isotonic or Isometric Exercise: Which Will Help You Most? | Forma Gym. https://formagym.com/isotonic-or-isometric-exercis e-which-will-help-you-most/

41 Andrew Payne (2021). Sagittal, Frontal and Transverse Plane: Movements and Exercises. https://blog.nasm.org/exercise-programming/sagittal-fronta l-traverse-planes-explained-with-exercises

42 Mansfield, P. (2019). *Essentials of Kinesiology for the Physical Therapist Assistant (Third Edition)* (3rd ed.). Mosby.

43 Valter Santilli, M. (2021). Clinical definition of sarcopenia. https://www. ncbi.nlm.nih.gov/pmc/articles/PMC4269139

44 Gahl, W. (2021). Mitochondria. https://www.genome.gov/genetics-glossary/ Mitochondria

45 https://www2.nau.edu/lrm22/lessons/atp/atp.html

46 Muscular Hypertrophy: The Science and Steps for Building Muscle. (2021). https://www.healthline.com/health/muscular-hypertrophy

47 Fast and Slow Twitch Muscle Fiber Types. (2021). https://www.verywellfit. com/fast-and- slow-twitch-muscle-fibers-3120094

48 https://www.nfpt.com/blog/proper-squat-training-personal-trainers

49 https://www.health.harvard.edu/staying-healthy/slowing-bone-loss-with-weight-bearing-exercise

Chapter 5

50 Roosevelt, T. (1899). Roosevelt, Theodore. 1900. The Strenuous Life; Essays and Addresses: I. The Strenuous Life. Retrieved from https://www.bartleby.com/58/1.html
51 Thayer, William Roscoe. *Theodore Roosevelt: An Intimate Biography.* Indybublish.com, 2008.
52 https://www.history.com/news/shot-in-the-chest-100-years-ago-teddy-roosevelt-kept-on-talking
53 Manners, W. *R and Will; a friendship that split the Republican Party.* New York: Harcourt, Brace & World, 1969.
54 www.eparmedx.com. (2019). *The Physical Activity Readiness Questionnaire for Everyone* (Ebook). http://eparmedx.com/wp-content/uploads/2013/03/FINAL-FILLABLE-ParQ-Plus-Jan-2019.pdf
55 Strength training: Get stronger, leaner, healthier. (2021). https://www.mayoclinic.org/healthy-lifestyle/fitness/in-depth/strength-training/art-20046670
56 Nast, C. (2021). The Only 7 Moves You Need to Get Strong as Hell. https://www.self.com/story/8-strength-exercises
57 Warner, J. (2021). Fitness Level Declines Dramatically with Age. https://www.webmd.com/fitness-exercise/news/ 20050725/fitness-level-declines-dramatically-with-age#1
58 ACE | Certified Personal Trainer | ACE Personal Trainer. (2021). https://www.acefitness.org/
59 LIVESTRONG.COM - Simple Healthy Living. (2021). https://www.livestrong.com/
60 https://www.nfpt.com/blog/gluteal-dysfunction
61 https://www.spine-health.com/conditions/sacroiliac-joint-dysfunction/sacroiliac-joint-dysfunction-symptoms-and-causes
62 https:// pubmed.ncbi.nlm.nih.gov/32132843/

Chapter 6

63 https://style.gq.com.qu/media/file_uploads/3/2/8/032835-1.jpg
64 https://www.nydailynews.com/life-style/health/hot-new-workout-sexercise-article-1.1592847

65 https://www.health.harvard.edu/healthbeat/is-sex-exercise-and-is-it-hard-on-the-heart

66 https://www.gq.com.au/fitness/workout/how-to-train-for-sex/news-story/8108b1c6eda2f71be7249d7489efecea

67 https://www.bodyand soul.com.au

68 https:www.health.harvard.edu/heartbeat/is-sex-exercise-and-is-it-hard-on-the-heart

69 https:www.yourhormones.info/hormones/testosterone/

70 Jackson G. Erectile dysfunction and cardiovascular disease. Arab J Urol. 2013 Sep;11(3):212-6. doi: 10.1016/j.aju.2013.03.003. Epub 2013 May 3. PMID: 26558084; PMCID: PMC4442980.

71 Jiannine LM. An investigation of the relationship between physical fitness, self-concept, and sexual functioning. J Educ Health Promot. 2018 May 3;7:57.doi: 10.4103/jehp.jehp_157_17. http://www.ncbi.nlm.nih.gov/pmc/articles/PMC5963212

72 Meldrum D.R., Gambone J.C., Morris M.A. A multifaceted approach to maximize erectile function and vascular health. *Fertil Steril.* 2010;947:2514–2520. Meldrum D.R., Gambone J.C., Morris M.A. Lifestyle and metabolic approaches to maximizing erectile and vascular health. *Int J Impot Res.* 2012;242:61–68.

73 Gerbild H, Larsen CM, Graugaard C, Areskoug Josefsson K. Physical Activity to Improve Erectile Function: A Systematic Review of Intervention Studies. Sex Med. 2018 Jun;6(2):75–89. doi: 10.1016/j.esxm.2018.02.001. Epub 2018 Apr 13. PMID: 29661646; PMCID: PMC5960035.

74 Lorenz TA, Meston CM. Acute exercise improves physical sexual arousal in women taking antidepressants. Ann Behav Med. 2012 Jun;43(3):352-61. doi: 10.1007/s12160-011-9338-1. PMID: 22403029; PMCID: PMC3422071.

75 Jiannine LM. An investigation of the relationship between physical fitness, self-concept, and sexual functioning. J Educ Health Promot. 2018 May 3;7:57. doi: 10.4103/jehp.jehp_157_17. PMID: 29922686; PMCID: PMC5963213.

76 Nancy Shute, "Is Sex Once a Week Enough for a Happy Relationship?" NPR, November 18,2015. https://www.tpr.org/science-technology/2015-11-18/is-sex-once-a-week-enough-for-a-happy-relationship

77 *Help Clients Overcome Plateaus and Manage Training Overloads.* National Federation of Professional Trainers. https://www.nfpt.com/blog/overcome-plateaus-and-training-overloads.

78 https://www.cdc.gov/nutrition/

79 https://health.gov/sites/default/files/2019-09/2015-2020_Dietary_
Guidelines.pdf

80 Ryu M.S., Aydemir TB. Zinc. In: Marriott BP, Birt DF, Stallings VA,
Yates AA, eds. Present Knowledge in Nutrition. 11ᵗʰ ed. Cambridge,
Massachusetts: Wiley-Blackwell; 2020:393-408.

81 Spencer H, Norris C, Williams D. Inhibitory effects of zinc on magnesium
balance and magnesium absorption in man. J Am Coll Nutr . 1994
Oct;13(5):479-84. doi: 10.1080/07315724.1994.1071843

82 Brisebois M, Kramer S, Lindsay KG, Wu CT, Kamla J. Dietary practices
and supplement use among CrossFit® participants. J Int Soc Sports Nutr.
2022 Jul 4;19(1):316-335. doi: 10.1080/15502783.2022.2086016. PMID:
35813850; PMCID: PMC9261745.

83 Kjekshus J. Inflammation: Friend and Foe. EBioMedicine. 2015 Jun
3;2(7):634-5. doi: 10.1016/j.ebiom.2015.05.029. PMID: 26288833;
PMCID: PMC4534693.

84 https://www.nutri-facts.org/en_US/home.html

85 Stecker RA, et. Al. Timing of erogenic aids and micronutrients on muscle and
exercise performance. J Int Soc Sports Nutr. 2019 Sep 2;16(1):37.doi:10.1186/
s12970-019-0304-9. PMID:31477133;PMCID:PMC6721335.

86 Torquati L, Peeters G, Brown WJ, Skinner TL. A Daily Cup of Tea or
Coffee May Keep You Moving: Association between Tea and Coffee
Consumption and Physical Activity. Int J Environ Res Public Health.
2018 Aug 22;15(9):1812. doi: 10.3390/ijerph15091812. PMID: 30135386;
PMCID: PMC6163361.

87 https:// www.medicinenet/how_bad_is_sodium_nitrate_ for_you/article.
htm.

88 Woessner, Mary, McIlvenna, Luke, Ortiz de Zevallos, Joaquin, Neil,
Christopher and Allen, Jason (2018) Dietary nitrate supplementation in
cardiovascular health: An ergogenic aid or exercise therapeutic? American
Journal of Physiology - Heart and Circulatory Physiology, 314 (2). H195 -
H212. ISSN 0363-6135

89 https://www. fortunebusinessinsights.com

90 Sztretye M, Dienes B, Gönczi M, Czirják T, Csernoch L, Dux L, Szentesi
P, Keller-Pintér A. Astaxanthin: A Potential Mitochondrial-Targeted
Antioxidant Treatment in Diseases and with Aging. Oxid Med Cell
Longev. 2019 Nov 11;2019:3849692. doi: 10.1155/2019/3849692. PMID:
31814873; PMCID: PMC6878783.

91 Matthew Walker, Why We Sleep: Unlocking the Power of Sleep and
Dreams. New York: Scribner, 2018.

92 https://www.dictionary.com

93 https://www.thehormonecurebook.com/

94 Massimo Bracci, et. al. Nocturnin Gene Diurnal Variation in Healthy Volunteers and Expression Levels in Shift Workers. Biomed Res Int, 2019, Jul 31. Doi:10.1155/2019/7582734 https://www.ncbi.nlm.nih.gov/pmc/articles/PMC6699378/#:~:text=The%20NOCTURNIN%20gene%20regulates%20the,alterations%20%5B5%E2%80%937%5D.

95 https://www.thensf.org/

96 https://www.nhlbi.nih.gov/files/docs/public/sleep/healthy_sleep.pdf

97 https://www.cdc.gov/bloodpressure/sleep.htm

98 https://www.thehormonecurebook.com/

99 Tim Ferriss. Tools of Titans. The Tactics, Routines, and Habits of Billionaires, Icons, and world-class Performers. New York, New York., Houghton Mifflin Harcourt Publishing Company, 2017.

100 https://www.hopkinsmedicine.org/health/wellness-and-prevention/choosing-the-best-sleep-position

101 https://www.thereadyspace.com

102 https://nfpt.com/blog/integrating-sleep-exercise-mutual-improvements

103 https://www.alekssalkin.com

104 https://www.mayoclinic.org.healthy-lifestyle/fitness/in-depth/strength-training/art-20046031

105 https://www.mrjamesnestor.com/breath

106 https: //www. Dossett,ML, Yeh, GY. Homeopathy Use in the United States and Implications for Public Health: A Review. Homeopathy. 2018 Feb; 107(1):3-9. doi: 10.1055/s-0037-1609016. Epub 2017 Dec 22. PMID:29528473;PMCID: PMC5989719.

107 https://www.medicalxpress.com/news/2016-02-survey-   american s-satisfaction-homeopathic-medicines.html

108 https://www.amalaims.org/homeopathyorgin.php

109 Wang S, Liu HY, Cheng YC, Su CH. Exercise Dosage in Reducing the Risk of Dementia Development: Mode, Duration, and Intensity-A Narrative Review. Int J Environ Res Public Health. 2021 Dec 17;18(24):13331. doi: 10.3390/ijerph182413331. PMID: 34948942; PMCID: PMC8703896.

110 Wang S, et.al. 2021.

111 https://accelerate.uofuhealth.utah.edu/resilience/neuroplasticity-how-to-use-your-brain-s-malleability-to-improve-your-well-being.

112 Admiral William H. McRaven (retired). *Make Your Bed: Little Things That Can Change Your Life … And Maybe the World.* New York: Grand Central Publishing (2017).

113 Michael F. Roisen, MD & Mehmet C. Oz, MD. You, Staying Young: The Owner's Manual for Extending Your Warranty. Waterville, ME: Thorndike Press, 2022.

Chapter 9

114 Ryan Denison. 2021. *"Nunc Coepi"*: The phrase that helped quarterback Philip Rivers persevere in faith, family, and football. https://www.denisonforum. org/ columns/sports/nunc-coepi-the-phrase-that-helped- quarterbac k-philip-rivers-persevere-in-faith-family- and-football/

Made in the USA
Las Vegas, NV
03 March 2024

86659567R00166